MY JOURNEY THROUGH THYROID CANCER AND OUT THE OTHER SIDE

GLENDA SHEPHERD

Dedicated to my husband Phil, who has given me unconditional love and support in the darkest times. Also dedicated to my surgeons and oncologist – you know who you are!

Contents

INTRODUCTION

Thyroid cancer is an unusual cancer, but fortunately often a very treatable one. Nobody really knows what causes it. As it affects mostly women, one theory is that the sudden weight gain and weight loss during pregnancy precipitates it, but there is also the theory that radiation to the face and neck during childhood (for example dental x-rays) may be a factor, and also some say the fallout from Chernobyl could be a cause. Incidences are rising. GP's only get to see one or two cases per year, so they are not always very knowledgeable on treatment procedures.

Anyone newly-diagnosed with thyroid cancer will find only some specialist hospitals can treat it (for example the hospital where I work does not treat it, and the oncologist there does not know much about it). They will also find that treatment procedures vary up and down the country. In some areas patients are offered multiple radioactive iodine (RAI) treatments, but patients in other areas are not. Some patients are given tracer scans with a very low dose of radioactive iodine before treatment is given, to see whether there is any uptake of radiation in the thyroid tissue, so in theory making sure that the thyroid tissue is receptive to the larger dose of radiation to come. Others are not offered a tracer scan, as another theory is that it stuns the thyroid cells and does not make them as receptive to the actual therapeutic dose of RAI and prolongs the treatment. There can also be differences of opinion on how long a patient is left on the T3 fast-acting liothyronine sodium before he or she is given the slower-releasing T4 levothyroxine tablets that they will take for life.

I have been supported over the years through being a member of the British Thyroid Foundation (http://www.btf-thyroid.org/) where you can find not only information regarding thyroid cancer, but also details on many other thyroid disorders (for example hypo/hyperthyroidism).

I hope this book is informative for anyone just diagnosed with thyroid cancer. I suppose we have the 'best' sort of cancer you can get, as survival rates are usually around 95%. I have heard it said that thyroid cancer is not really a cancer, but unfortunately it certainly is and what is more may prove fatal if not treated, as there might be spread to the lungs and/or bones. The treatment is radical, just the same as for any other cancer, and the after-effects of treatment are lifelong.

Please do not expect this story to be a walk in the park; the procedures and operations I had to undergo left its mark on me in many ways. However, I am still here and fortunately have found a way of living with thyroid cancer. They say everyone has a story to tell. I did not for a moment expect mine to be this one.

This book incorporates books 1, 2 and 3 in the 'Living With Thyroid Cancer' series. There are also updates in 2019 as to my condition now, and extra information regarding the legacy of thyroid cancer and how you might feel after you have been through the same journey as I have.

Perhaps he knew, as I did not, that the Earth was made round so that we would not see too far down the road.

Karen Blixen

CHAPTER 1 – THE START OF IT ALL

On the Isle of Wight's Sandown beach in October 2004, I stood barefoot with my husband, Phil, at the water's edge. Looking back across the beach, I spotted Phil's sister Mary and her husband Dave wrapped up in towels on their sunbeds to protect them from the cold wind that had suddenly sprung up. Dave and his camera were never too far away from each other, and I heard him calling to us to pose for a photo. He walked over to us, camera in hand, and said something silly to make us laugh whilst he snapped away.

The four of us were on a long weekend break staying at a bungalow in Bembridge owned by Dave's sister Betty. We had all had a pretty good year thus far; we had attended the wedding of our eldest son Lee to Sarah on a glorious day in May, and Mary and Dave had recently announced a third grandchild was on the way. Phil and I were due to become grandparents the following July as Sarah was newly pregnant. We were also looking forward to another long weekend break together at the Center Parcs holiday village in Elveden, Suffolk, in December, about a half hour drive from our home. The short break would not only be with Mary, Dave and their daughter Jenny, but also Lee and Sarah were coming along and our youngest son Matthew and his girlfriend Anna.

We often met up with Mary and Dave, and we had all married

within a week of each other early in October 1980. We originally lived near to them in Croydon, Surrey, where Phil had been born and brought up, but moved to a village near Bury St Edmunds in 1991 due to Phil's new job being based in Palgrave, near Diss in Norfolk. Problems had arisen when it was taking him three hours to travel to Palgrave from Croydon, and usually longer than that to travel home every night. We had two young sons and welcomed taking them out of the London suburbs and living the country life. After the first year of adjustment to the slower pace of life we were now fully-fledged country folk. After 13 years of living the country life, we had no plans to ever move back to London.

***

What we were all unaware of as we posed for that photo on Sandown beach, was that before a month had gone by Dave was to suffer a heart attack (which luckily he recovered from after treatment), and I was to find a lump in my neck whilst putting on a necklace. Nobody knows what fate has in store. I read somewhere that the world was made round so we don't see too far down the road. Perhaps that's just as well.

I had no idea how long the lump had been there. The oncologist I saw a few months into the treatment said it could have been there for years. The neck area is not a place where you're told to check for lumps. Leaflets picked up in the GP surgery told me that I needed to be 'breast aware' and to have cervical smears every three years, but I'd never even considered the neck area when thinking about cancer – even though I've since found out that thyroid cancer affects mostly women. My father and his brother had both died of cancer at age 49, one of prostate cancer and the other of a brain tumour. My mother contracted cancer of the uterus in her sixties, but survived after having a hysterectomy and radiotherapy (she is now in her eighties and living near me in warden-assisted sheltered housing). Two of my grandparents had also died in their seventies of cancer, one of pancreatic cancer, and the other of lung cancer (probably due to my grandfather being a heavy smoker though).

As I approached my forties I started to worry that maybe I too was at risk of cancer due to this unhealthy legacy. Also over the previous decade I had begun to put on weight, and suffered with terrible PMT symptoms. At about age 37 I was feeling so awful that I had to do something about it. I saw a gynaecologist who prescribed the mini-pill (Norethisterone) which miraculously took all my PMT symptoms away, and I began a long-overdue exercise programme.

Ten years on, at age 47, I was still jogging nearly every day before starting work at 7.30am as a ward clerk at my local hospital, rising at 5.15am to run a 2-mile circuit of our picturesque village. I enjoyed the early morning sunrises and the feeling that the village was mine alone as I pounded the pavements when everyone else was in bed. I ate a low-fat diet to keep my weight down; indeed since being pregnant with Matthew in 1985 I could not stomach any fried or fatty foods anyway, as they would instantly make me feel nauseous. In my early forties I had also started to feel sick if I had cow's milk in tea (a skin test confirmed a milk intolerance), and cheese and chocolate which previously I had eaten with abandon started off migraines, so I had switched to soya milk, which luckily I preferred the taste of in tea (de-caffeinated of course!). From being overweight and feeling miserable and eating lots of unhealthy foods in my thirties, I was now the veritable picture of health. The only problem I had started to suffer with was a locking jaw at night. I had no idea why the jaw locked whilst I was asleep – the dentist said that it could be caused by the unconscious grinding of my teeth.

I decided to make an appointment with the GP about the lump in my neck but was not overly worried; it was probably a pulled muscle due to all the neck exercises I did to keep the ravages of time at bay.

The end of November 2004 saw me waiting in the GP surgery. The doctor felt my neck and noted that the lump moved when I swallowed. She wanted to refer me to a consultant endocrinologist at the hospital where I worked, as she thought I had a cyst on my thyroid. The thyroid is a butterfly-shaped gland at the front of the neck which secretes the hormone Thyroxine, and this has an effect on the body's metabolic rate (how quickly you burn up food). As I was included on Phil's medical insurance policy and wanted to be seen sooner rather than later, I let the GP know I would like to be seen privately at the Nuffield hospital in Bury St Edmunds. I completed the paperwork required and waited for an appointment to arrive through the post.

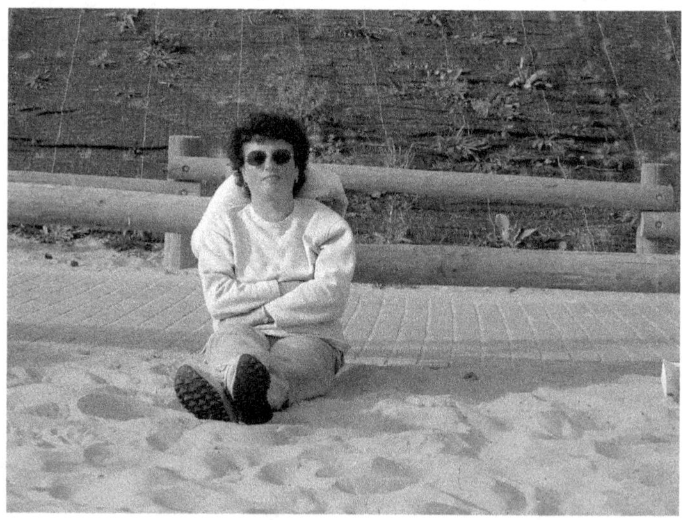

The lump seems quite visible here on a Center Parcs holiday in August 2003, but surprisingly enough I never noticed it until over a year later.

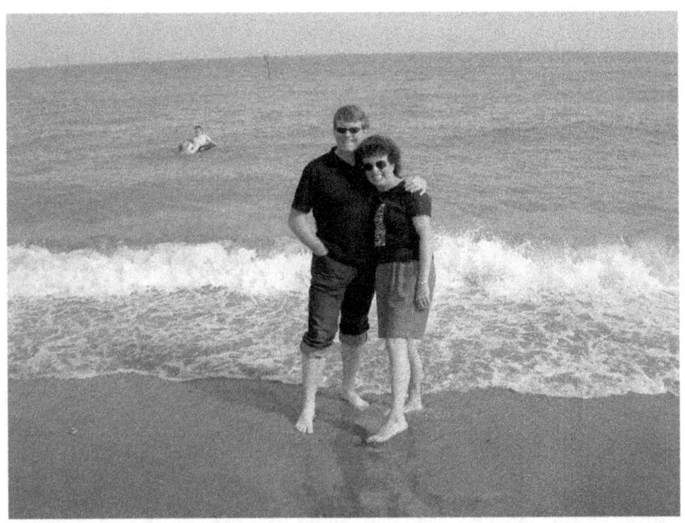

Photo shows Phil and me on the beach at Sandown, Isle of Wight. October 2004. Dave's saying something to make us laugh, but I can't remember what.

CHAPTER 2 – EARLY YEARS

I was born Glenda Ann Wood on October 28th 1957, and spent my early childhood living in the East London suburb of Poplar, with my parents. Originally we had lived in a large (and haunted) flat above what used to be Barclays Bank at 819 Commercial Road, Poplar (the flat is still there, but the bank is now a café).

I was aware at a very young age of a strange presence in the flat; my bedroom was always colder than the rest of the house, and I often saw the ghosts of animals in the hallway. My mother once told me of an occasion where I was staying overnight with my grandmother, but the imprint of a body in my bed still remained even though the bed had been tidied the previous day and nobody had slept in it. I remember as a very young child that sometimes my bed would shake uncontrollably and I would dive under the covers in fright, hoping the shaking would go away. I had no idea what caused it, and over a period of time accepted it as 'normal'. The psychic phenomena I experienced as a young child in the flat started my lifelong interest in the spirit world.

My parents rented the flat at a reduced rate as my father was a bank employee (or maybe it was cheap because of the other-wordly presence?). Years later I found out that somebody had committed suicide in the flat. It was no place for a young child of five to live in though, as there were no children nearby to play with, and I was too young and the streets below far too busy for me to play outside. I had no siblings, and had started to play with imaginary friends.

My parents wanted a home in a quieter location away from the constant heavy traffic rumbling past outside, and from the undesirables that often slept on the main doorstep downstairs that led out onto the Commercial Road. They also wanted to move me from Mayflower Primary School in Upper North Street, as I was not enjoying the experience (to put it mildly). The council found us a prefabricated home a mile or so away at number 3 Layfield Place (off Byron Street, but alas no longer there) that was supposed to have been only temporary whilst we waited for permanent accommodation. The 'temporary' wait eventually stretched to seven years!

The 'prefab' as far as I was concerned, was idyllic. I much preferred it to the flat in Commercial Road, as we were on the ground floor and I could play in our sizeable garden. The psychic happenings disappeared, and were only to surface very infrequently from then on. I found a couple of 'best' friends who lived nearby, and attended a new school, Manorfield Primary, in St. Leonard's road, where my fledgling musical talents were encouraged by the formidable Miss Anderson. I began to play the violin, but the road to perfection was long (after an evening sawing away, I found that Dad had 'accidentally' trodden on the violin the next morning!).

At age 11 I attended George Green Grammar School in the East India Dock Road. My fondest memories of that school were throwing left-overs from my lunch down to the boys' playground on the street level from the girls' playground up on the roof, and hoping to score a direct hit on one of the more obnoxious boys in the process who constantly made fun of my wild, curly hair. When going home from school I had to walk through Crisp Street with all its shops and market stalls, and I can still hear all the market traders' calls in my head. My favourite stall was the old 45rpm record stall. Most of my pocket money was blown on rock n' roll records, comics, sweets, and

Enid Blyton books bought from Segal's bookshop (my favourite shop but alas no longer there) on the East India Dock Road .

My childhood years were very happy and I had total freedom to roam the streets with friends, something I would not have let my own children do if they had been brought up in the same part of London today, as it has now totally changed as you can imagine. We explored condemned houses that were due to be demolished to make way for the A102M motorway, played 'Knock Down Ginger' in Balfron Towers, and scared ourselves silly playing 'Chicken' down by the Blackwall Tunnel. Mum and Dad were not on the end of a mobile phone, and if we got into scrapes, then we had to get out of them ourselves. When our prefab home (and in fact Layfield Place itself) was due to be demolished to make way for what is now a technical college, the council had no choice but to re-house us. We moved across the river and I suddenly had to leave behind all that was familiar when I was 13 (the photo below shows me aged about 10 with my parents).

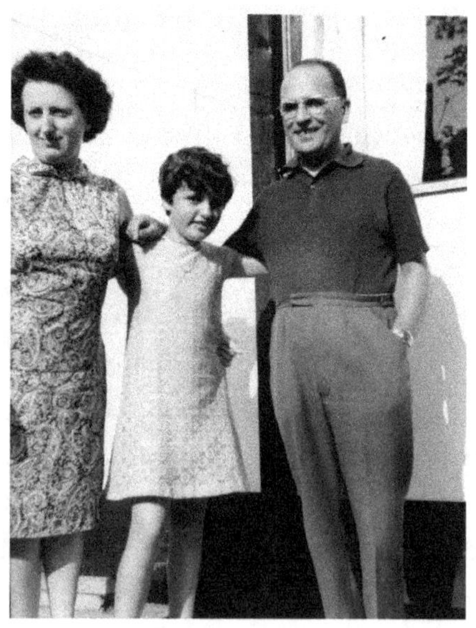

My teenage years were spent living in Kidbrooke, South East London, on a huge sprawling council estate that is now thankfully in the process of being demolished. I loathed the estate as soon as I saw it, and my opinion never changed in the seven or so years that I lived there. I was content though with my new school, Kidbrooke Comprehensive (the same school that latterly Jamie Oliver trialled with the new healthy school meals), after the initial strangeness had worn off. I had a few very good friends, and took part with them in virtually all extra-curricular musical activities. I left school in 1976 and went to work as a laboratory technician for a company that has now been taken over by GlaxoSmithKline. The following year, when I was 19, my father died of cancer of the prostate which had spread to his bones. He had contracted cancer at the age of 47; the same age as I had been when I found the lump in my neck. I helped my mother to organise his funeral, but due to my young age I realise with hindsight that I was not much of a comfort to her in the months afterwards.

I knew by the age of 20 that I wanted to leave home to forge a life of my own, as my late nights (due to my increasingly regular attendance at various local discotheques) were having an unfortunate effect on my mother's sleeping habits (what goes around comes around, and it would be me waiting at the top of the stairs 25 years later as Lee crept up at 4am after a night out on the lash). I rented a flat in Anerley near Crystal Palace with a workmate. It certainly helped both of us as my mother then aged 54, after finding herself living alone for the first time in 25 years, learned to drive, drove herself and friends to various local dances, and even in time found a boyfriend. I quickly learnt to look after myself, cook, and do small repair jobs on my car. Myself and my flatmate had the time of our lives whilst living in our little attic flat, staying out dancing until late, giving parties, and falling in love with undesirable work colleagues, all the things you do when you're young and silly!

Whilst living at the flat in Anerley, I met the man who was to be my husband. Phil had also come from a huge council estate in New Addington, Croydon and had lots of siblings, something I envied him for, having always wanted a sister or brother of my own. We became engaged three months after meeting, and married on October 11th 1980 in St. James Church, Kidbrooke. In the same month I left my job due to various allergies to workplace conditions, and became a library assistant at Anerley library near to my old attic flat in Waldegrave Road. We went on to have two sons, Lee, born in July 1982, and Matthew, born in November 1985. Life was good. I had a lovely husband, two sons to love and care for, and we now had a home of our own in Addiscome near Croydon, albeit with a mortgage up to the hilt.

I stayed at home for 12 years looking after the boys, which had its rewards as well as its down moments. During that time we moved from London to a village near Bury St Edmunds to be closer to Phil's workplace, and also to give the boys a better life. When Lee was 12 and Matthew was 8 I started back at work as an office clerk for a small company dealing in the sales of lime and fertiliser to the farmer. It had taken me three years of applying for jobs to secure the post, and I was beginning to think that at the age of 36 and with two young children I would never work again. I am very determined though, and vowed I would not give up until I did get a job. I carried on over the next 10 years through two other administration jobs ending up working as a ward clerk at my local hospital in Bury St Edmunds, and all the time applying for higher-grade administrative vacancies in the NHS which sadly seemed very elusive. I did not mind working as a ward clerk though, but was ever hopeful that something better would be just around the corner. Unfortunately it would be something worse around the corner and it was coming straight at me …

CHAPTER 3 – VISIT TO THE ENDOCRINOLOGIST & 1ST SCAN

The appointment date to see the consultant endocrinologist was not long in arriving. I went to see him in early December 2004 at his private clinic at the Nuffield hospital. He explained that the lump probably was a cyst, but would take some blood to check if the thyroid was working properly, and there would be more blood tests and a 24-hour urine test also to determine whether cancer was present, but he stressed that the lump probably was not cancerous at all as there was no history of thyroid cancer in my family. I was told that I would also need an ultrasound scan and possibly a needle biopsy of the cyst at the same time. I explained I would soon be on a long weekend break at Center Parcs and he said he would speak to the consultant radiologist to ensure I had the scan before I went. He said it was also a good idea to get a sample of blood to see if I was at the menopause. I was to come back and see him near the end of December for the results.

His nurse took the blood tests there and then, and I was sent home with two large plastic urine collection bottles. He explained that as I was at work during the week, it would be best to wait for a Sunday to fill the urine bottles as it would be more convenient than having to carry them about at work all day! I agreed totally, and spent the next Sunday dutifully filling the bottles ready to take to

Pathology on the Monday morning when I went back to work.

We were due for our Center Parcs visit on the 10th December, and on the 9th I had my ultrasound scan in the X-Ray Department at the Nuffield. The consultant radiologist could see my thyroid was covered in cysts. He said he was not worried as the whole thyroid was lumpy rather than just one piece of it. He said he was not even going to take a needle biopsy, as the result would just come back as benign cells. I was reassured when he said nothing needed to be done other than regular check-ups to see if the cyst had grown any bigger. He would report back to the endocrinologist, and I would get his report and the results of the blood tests when I had my second endocrinology appointment just before Christmas. He thought it was a multinodular goitre (looking back with hindsight, it would have been a good idea at that point to seek a second opinion!).

Meanwhile there was Center Parcs to enjoy. Myself and Phil, Lee now aged 22 and his new wife Sarah, plus Matthew aged 19 and girlfriend Anna met up with Mary, Dave, and Jenny. We had adjoining chalets and everyone was set to have a good time. We had all been visiting Center Parcs since the boys and Jenny were small. Dave had recently had to have one of his arteries opened up with a stent. The artery had become clogged over the years, which had given him the mild heart attack a couple of months before. He looked pale and seemed more tired than usual, but was still cracking jokes and making people laugh. He did not fancy playing Badminton which he had done in the past (which was a shame as he is so bad at it that it's hysterical to watch), but to my surprise put on a pair of roller skates and skated around the rink with the rest of us. We could not believe he had been in the Coronary Care Unit only a short while before, and now here he was balancing on a pair of skates. He had been told by his cardiologist to change his diet to a low-fat one which meant cutting out his beloved cheese, but other than that was set to lead a normal life.

Center Parcs turned out to be not so much fun as it had been in previous years when the boys and Jenny were small. I was still thinking about the lump in my neck and what the blood tests would reveal. Dave was tired and not as jolly as he used to be (understandable due to what he had undergone), and there was also some friction between a few of the young people, which also affected us and Mary and Dave. Unhappily the holiday ended on a rather sour note, and I think everyone was pleased to go home on the last day.

Left to right, Lee, Sarah, Jenny, Matt, Anna,
and myself at Center Parcs Dec 04

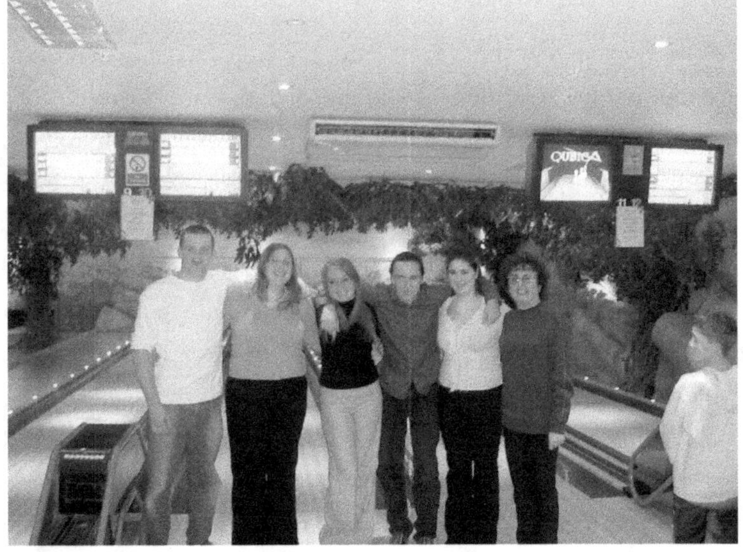

Phil and I skating at Center Parcs December 2004.

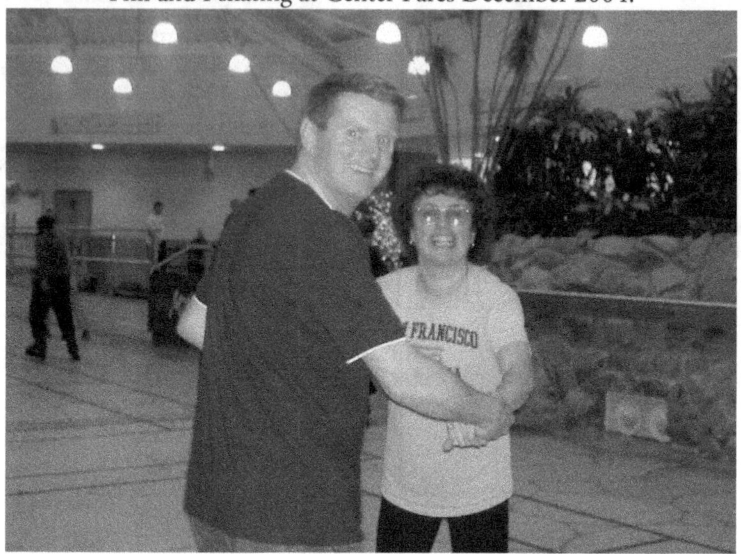

A week or so after the Center Parcs break, it was time to return to the endocrinologist at the Nuffield Hospital to learn the results of all the tests. He was most encouraging. He told me my thyroid was working normally, that the blood and urine tests were clear – indeed I had lovely 'rich' blood. He diagnosed a multinodular goitre (I suppose he was basing his findings on the ultrasound report) and told me I would need only regular scans to keep an eye on the cyst to check it wasn't getting any bigger. If it was not causing me any problems he suggested leaving it alone.

The only cloud on the horizon was that he was unable to determine if I was menopausal. Apparently the norethisterone tablets which I had been taking for ten years to combat the dreadful symptoms of pre-menstrual tension were keeping my follicle stimulating hormone and luteinising hormone levels artificially low (if I had been menopausal the levels would have been sky-high). In order to obtain a blood sample that wasn't affected by the tablets, I would have to come off them for at least three months and then have another blood test. I could do that I thought – that was easy. What with my healthy eating I probably wouldn't have the symptoms now anyway. I made an appointment for March 29th to have another check-up scan and then I positively skipped out of the hospital – now I could enjoy Christmas with my family.

We usually treat ourselves and have Christmas day lunch out at a restaurant. That year it was at the Rushbrooke Arms in Bury St Edmunds with Phil, Matt, Anna and my mother. A New Year's Eve dinner and dance at The Quality Hotel in Norwich was planned with Phil, Lee and Sarah (ever-expanding with our first grandchild), and Matt and Anna. We stayed overnight at the hotel and all had an enjoyable time. We usually saw Mary and Dave over the Christmas period but this year they had other plans (I think the disappointing Center Parcs holiday still loomed large in everyone's minds).

New Year's Eve dinner at The Quality Hotel, Norwich.
Left side from the front, myself, Phil, and Anna.
Right side from the front, Lee, Sarah, and Matt.

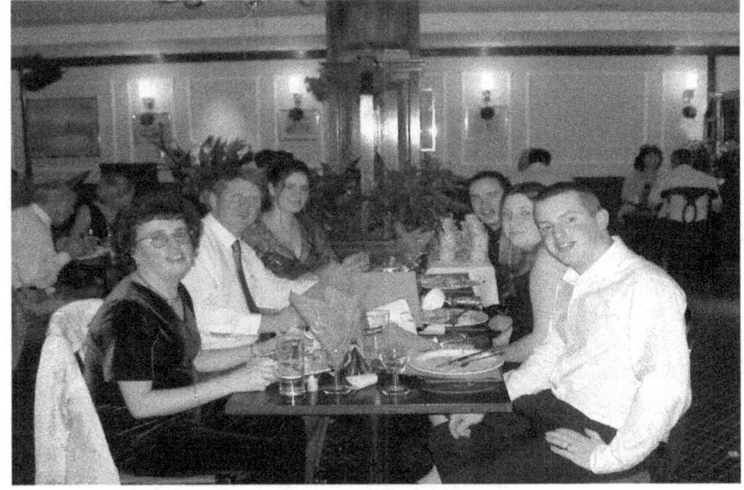

CHAPTER 4 – VISIT TO THE ENDOCRINOLOGIST & 2ND SCAN

January and February 2005 passed in the usual whirlwind of work, eat, and sleep. I was also organising quite a few gigs for Matt's heavy rock band and we were often out weekends until the early hours at gigs in London and the South East. Phil and I had grown up in the Seventies' listening to loud rock bands, and it was with a certain amount of relief when Matt mastered the intricacies of the electric guitar and veered towards the music we loved instead of the (as far as I'm concerned) terrible house, garage, trance, dance, rap/crap genres that Lee had favoured as a teenager and had us reaching in for the earplugs. Funnily enough though, as Lee has got older he plays rock music in his van all day, so perhaps some of our tastes did rub off on him after all.

I kept a close watch on the cyst during January and February to see if it was getting any bigger. Towards the end of February I thought that it had increased in size a little bit, but decided the scan in March would show if it had. I felt ok. I'd had no real PMT symptoms either. Thank goodness I can come off the tablets now I thought, because it must be the healthy eating that had altered my body chemistry.

By the time the scan was due at the end of March, I knew the cyst was bigger. I could feel it in my neck as it started to cause a little pressure. I was often getting choking feelings and had to keep coughing, especially if I laid on my left side. I mentioned all this to the radiologist who again performed the scan, and he said it had increased only marginally. I mentioned it again at the next appointment with the endocrinologist on April 11th where I was to be told the result of the latest scan. He surprisingly said that although the radiologist had told him verbally that the cyst was bigger, he hadn't actually written the fact on his report.

The endocrinologist asked me what I wanted to do about the cyst. He said if it continued growing, it would possibly interfere with my swallowing and breathing mechanisms. I had already decided upon surgery to remove it before the appointment, after having had a surprise telephone conversation with my aunt a week or so previously. The end result being I was to be referred to a consultant endocrine surgeon who would remove the cyst surgically at the Nuffield in Bury St Edmunds in the near future.

I had found out, whilst speaking on the phone to my aunt in March, that she had had a cyst on her thyroid removed about ten years previously. I had not been aware of this, as we did not see each other very often. She had told me her cyst had been the size of a fist and had spread down into her chest, but had not been cancerous. Doctors had taken half of her thyroid gland away in order to remove the cyst, but apart from recently having to start taking Thyroxine tablets because of excessive tiredness, she was now feeling fine. She also thought her own mother had had thyroid problems which were never treated during her lifetime. I realised that thyroid disease probably ran in my father's side of the family and I that I had probably inherited the onerous trait.

The endocrinologist also enquired how it had been for me coming off the norethisterone tablets in December. I mentioned the two symptom-free periods which occurred in January and February, but so far at the end of March no period had arrived. He said it was common to miss periods when coming off long-term use of hormone tablets.

My periods still had not returned by May 3rd, the date of the surgeon's appointment. I wondered how long I would have waited on the NHS to be seen, and thanked my lucky stars that I was covered by medical insurance. I sat and faced the surgeon on that Tuesday morning, and he explained that it was too dangerous to undertake a partial thyroidectomy. If in later years the remaining thyroid gland also needed to be removed, there would have been too much scar tissue in place from the first operation, and the surgeon would have had trouble seeing what he was doing with this in the way. He told me that the operation would be a total thyroidectomy and that it was a major operation, possibly taking about three hours to perform. His duty was also to tell me of the possible damage to the nerves controlling the vocal cords as he would have to be working quite near the voice box, and of the inadvertent removal of the parathyroid glands during the operation, which control calcium metabolism. He reassured me that he was experienced at thyroid removals and his patients did not often suffer these consequences, but it was his duty to ensure I was fully informed of the dangers involved. He reassured me that he always took pains to find and trace the nerve to the voice box before removing the thyroid, and blood tests were taken soon after surgery to check the blood calcium levels which would start to drop if the parathyroid glands had been caught up in the removed thyroid tissue.

I decided I had no choice but to go ahead with the surgery. I realised the anaesthetist might have a problem with my locking jaw when he put me to sleep and tried to put the intubation tube down my throat to ventilate me before surgery. I mentioned this to the surgeon who said he would refer me to a consultant oral surgeon. I had never seen so many doctors in my life in the space of just a few months. All I had ever had were colds and coughs and the usual childhood illnesses, and now I was facing a major operation and possibly another one on my locking jaw.

Below are the original ultrasound scan reports showing that the radiologist felt no biopsy was needed as only an 'intra-cystic papilloma' (benign tumour) might possibly be found, and that on the second scan he had failed to mention the enlargement that had taken place. He had however mentioned it verbally to the endocrinologist.

6-NOV-2006 12:49   FROM:MMP   01223266927   TO:901284713183   P.1/2

Our Ref: RPB/AKB

23rd November 2004

Dr
The Bury St Edmunds Nuffield Hospital
St Marys Square
Bury St Edmunds
Suffolk
IP33 2AA

Dear Dr

Glenda Shepherd DOB 28.10.1957

ULTRASOUND THYROID   23.11.04   Reported 23.11.04

Both lobes of the thyroid show diffuse focal nodular change with cystic areas within. On the right side there is a relatively well defined cyst of approximately 5 mms with an obvious echogenic centre. The nature of this is unclear and may represent an old haemorrhage but obviously an intra-cystic papilloma cannot be excluded. The nodular change throughout the remainder of the right lobe of thyroid is evident. Within the left lobe in the upper pole there is extensive nodular change with obvious calcification within. In the lower pole on the left side extending into the isthmus there is some cystic areas. This would appear to be the palpable area.

In light of the above I think needling the lower aspect is not indicated and I think possibly trying to needle the right cystic lesion would be extremely difficult. Can we discuss with regard to further assessment?

Dr

29th March 2005

Consultant Physician
The Bury St Edmunds Nuffield Hospital
St Marys Square
Bury St Edmunds
Suffolk
IP33 2AA

Dear Dr

Glenda Shepherd DOB 28.10.1957

ULTRASOUND THYROID   29.03.05   Reported 29.03.05

The multi nodular changes around both lobes of the thyroid are again noted. I think there has been little significant change from previous examination. Could we please discuss further assessment?

Dr

CHAPTER 5 – APPOINTMENT WITH THE ORAL SURGEON

A couple of weeks after the appointment with the surgeon, I received a letter from the Nuffield hospital to say the date for my surgery was Monday June 13th 2005 and that I needed to attend the Pre-Admission Clinic on June 2nd. There was also an appointment for me to see the oral surgeon on June 7th for my jaw problems. Bliss and joy. The Pre-Admission nurse was kindness personified. I had nose and groin swabs to check I was not MRSA positive (as I worked in an NHS hospital, they were particularly worried about this, as the patients in the Nuffield all had their own rooms and MRSA was unheard of), and I had my blood pressure and heart rate checked, which because I was nervous was running a little high (I had begun to suffer from chronic white-coat syndrome!).

The in-house doctor took some blood, listened to my heart, asked me if I had any cracked teeth, and gave me an ECG which showed no problems. I mentioned a crack in a lower molar which caused pain if I chewed on any hard foodstuffs. The pain had been there for about 5 years and caused only intermittent problems, and the dentist had suggested leaving it alone. My temperature was normal. I had started a very heavy period on May 20th which was in its 14th day with no sign of stopping, so did not want to do a urine test. The nurse said not to worry as that could be done on the day of admission. I secretly hoped the period would be finished before then, as I didn't really want to have to cope with that as well. I made a mental note to give it one more month to see if things settled down and then resume the Norethisterone tablets if the periods were still haywire. I mentioned the locking jaw dysfunction, and the doctor said it could be a problem during the operation and he made a note of it.

I was starting to feel nervous about the operation. I had never had an anaesthetic or any sort of operation before. I had only been in hospital twice before, and each time had come out holding a baby. That was not going to happen this time. I wondered what the oral surgeon would say about the locking jaw. Perhaps he would stop the operation from going ahead?

The maxillo-facial (oral) surgeon felt all around my jaw and asked me to open and close my mouth. My mouth apparently pulled down to the right. He said the jaw was out of alignment, and he then sent me for an x-ray which revealed quite a bit of wear and tear on the left jaw joint, probably due to grinding my teeth whilst asleep. The result was I would need surgery to repair the left side of the jaw, but the operation on my thyroid could go ahead; the anaesthetist would just need to be careful when manipulating it. Meanwhile he said he would write to my dentist to instruct him to make me a night-time splint, which would solve the locking problem in the short-term. I knew I would never be able to sleep with any sort of device in my mouth, so discounted that solution immediately. He told me to make another appointment to see him when I wanted the surgery done. From 47 years with no medical problems to two operations needed probably only a few months apart, all my Christmases had come at once.

CHAPTER 6 - THE DAY OF THE THYROIDECTOMY

Phil drove me to the Nuffield hospital on the day of surgery. I likened it mentally to a drive to the executioner's chamber. I'd had nothing to eat or drink as requested and was feeling terribly nervous. My work colleagues had all wished me well and the ward manager had given me three weeks off to recuperate. I hoped that was all I needed.

I was shown to room 26 - a pleasant downstairs room with its own bath and toilet, and patio doors leading on to a communal garden. There was the usual hospital bed and call bells, but also carpet on the floor, an armchair, television, and chairs for visitors. Phil and I were told by a nurse that I was on the afternoon list for surgery, and during the morning would be seen by the in-house doctor and anaesthetist. I was disappointed to have to wait at least another five hours before surgery. I was feeling tired and shaky, through lack of sleep and food, and wanted it to be over with quickly. I was given menus to fill out for supper that night, and the following day's meals. The food sounded quite nice and I was eager to eat some of it. I mentioned that I did not eat dairy produce to the 'hostess' who came to collect the menus, and she said that would not be a problem; the chef could make my usual morning porridge with soya milk.

We settled down, resigned to the long wait. I tried to concentrate on a crossword puzzle book I had brought in, and Phil read the morning newspaper. Over the next few years he would become quite an expert at sitting in hospital rooms (a sixth sense told him what I required when I was wheeled back from various operations), but this was his first time as my little helper, apart from when I had had babies over 20 years previously. I could not settle, and opened the patio doors to go into the garden. It was peaceful; all the other patients were still in bed I assumed, and for a while I watched the birds feeding on the little bird table. I went into the bathroom and rinsed my mouth several times for something to do. The temptation to take a giant swig of water was almost too much. Phil would not eat or drink anything in front of me, so he stayed nil by mouth too.

We were left to our own devices for almost four hours. Towards lunchtime the anaesthetist came in. He listened to my chest, asked if I was allergic to any medications and if I had had a bad reaction in the past to any anaesthetics. I replied I knew of no medications I was allergic to, and that I had never had an anaesthetic before. I told him of the locking jaw problem and he noted it on the pink anaesthetic card. He told me I looked nervous and I assured him I was terrified.

Things started to move a bit after that. The doctor came in and prescribed some tranquilisers to settle me as he'd obviously communicated with the anaesthetist. The nurse put an ID wristband on me, measured me for stockings to combat DVT (blood clots forming in the legs due to being immobile), and told me to put on my hospital gown. Phil tied it up at the back and assured me my behind was not hanging out. Nurse came back with the stockings and put them on for me. They felt quite tight and she said they were very good at stopping blood clots forming, and that I could take them home afterwards to use on any long-haul airplane flight. We had a Caribbean cruise booked in November to celebrate our 25th wedding anniversary and I resolved to use them again then.

Nurse gave me the medications the doctor had prescribed, and also a pre-med to make me feel sleepy. I was told to get into bed, which I dutifully did. I stared at the ceiling and prayed for sleep but it did not come. Suddenly there was panic; the nurse appeared again and asked had I signed a consent form? I replied in the negative. Organised chaos ensued as the surgeon had to be found to give me the consent form and I had just been given heavy medication. A few moments later he appeared with the form for signing. I was still lucid when I signed it and still fully awake when the porter came to take me to the operating theatre just before 2 o'clock. Phil walked down with me, gave me a kiss, and said he would see me later. He probably then went off for some well-deserved lunch.

The anaesthetist greeted me inside the operating theatre, checked my wristband against his list of patients, and then began to put a cannula in my left hand. He good-naturedly complained that ladies' veins were always smaller. He then injected a liquid into the cannula and said it would make me feel sleepy. It certainly did, as I remember nothing after that until I woke up in the recovery room some three hours later. I was in a sitting position propped up with pillows instead of lying down, and the recovery room nurse assured me that now I was awake, I could be taken back to my room.

CHAPTER 7 – THE AFTERMATH OF THE THYROIDECTOMY

Feeling much relieved that it was all over, I was wheeled back to room 26. There was Phil sitting waiting patiently to tend to my every need, bless him. I felt wide awake and not at all sick. I'd heard the usual tales of patients being sick after surgery and resigned myself to the fact that it would probably happen to me. The anaesthetist had told me on his earlier visit that he always gave his patients a powerful anti-sickness drug through the cannula and I was pleased to say it was still working. There were devices on my lower legs that inflated and deflated at regular intervals, obviously helping out the stockings in their anti-DVT mission, and an oxygen tube going into my nose to oxygenate my red blood cells I was told.

I reached up to feel my neck but Phil gently took my arm and said not to touch the wound. I told him I needed a wee really badly. My voice came out as a whisper. Phil at first thought I was still circling the airport – how could I need a wee when I'd had nothing to drink since the day before? I repeated my need for the loo again and the nurse brought a bedpan. I was mortified but felt too weak to get up and go to the toilet. Phil and the nurse helped me on to it and I duly performed. It seemed only five minutes later when I needed another wee, and another wee after that. A stack of bedpans was hurriedly left in the room for my use. Fluids had been pumped through the cannula during the operation to keep me hydrated, and now they wanted to come out! I was piddling for England and also Ireland, Scotland and Wales for that matter. My little helper Phil became 'King of the Bedpan's, and did not flinch once in his duty.

My blood pressure, pulse and temperature were being closely monitored. The blood pressure and pulse were raised, but my temperature was normal. The nurse was concerned about how fast my heart rate was. I could feel it pounding away in my chest even though I was lying still. The Doctor was called and came and duly did an ECG, but he said he was not concerned as the beat was regular. Whilst raising my gown to attach the ECG electrodes, a rash appeared on my chest which mysteriously vanished again in seconds. It seemed I was having some sort of reaction to the anaesthetic or pre-med or both. In my befuddled state, I hoped I wasn't going to have a heart attack. The doctor went away, and observations continued to be taken at regular intervals by the nursing staff.

I came to the realisation that I felt terribly weak and seemed to have no voice or coughing mechanism to speak of. My heart was racing and I could not turn my head from side to side, as the stitches pulled in my neck. Not being able to cough properly was worrying as there suddenly seemed lots of phlegm on my chest that I was unable to shift which seemed to be getting stuck in the back of my throat. I could not believe I had gone from being reasonably fit to being struck down in a hospital bed hardly able to move within the space of a few hours.

More was to come. The surgeon appeared in my room after completing his afternoon operating list. He thought it best to tell me that he did not like the look of the thyroid gland that he had taken out. In his experience he thought it had looked possibly cancerous, and he had sent it away to the laboratory to be analysed. He had also taken out four lymph nodes in my neck which had been swollen, and these too would be tested for cancer.

I could not believe what I was hearing. It was like a bad dream that I could not wake up from. The radiologist had assured me the lump was just a cyst; the endocrinologist had told me it was ok to leave it alone if it wasn't causing problems, and now I was being told that the lump was probably cancerous. The radiologist had not even thought it was necessary to perform a needle biopsy of the lower left thyroid, which I found out later almost certainly would have detected the cancer present.

I did not doubt the surgeon at all; he had had enough experience to know a cancerous thyroid when he saw one. I realised I should have had surgery after the first ultrasound scan; how much could the cancer have spread in the intervening six months? The surgeon did add that thyroid cancer was easily treatable, and that my chances of survival would be in the region of 95 per cent. I would need radioactive iodine (RAI) at a later date to kill off any thyroid cells left in my body, and therefore kill the cancer contained within them. Thyroid cells are particularly partial to iodine (they need it to make the hormone thyroxine). After making any remaining thyroid cells sensitive to RAI by coming off the thyroxine tablets I would need to take and eating a low-iodine diet, the cells would then gobble up the RAI and be destroyed even if the cancer had spread elsewhere in the body (as any spread would be made up of thyroid cells). It sounded simple. I asked him where thyroid cancer usually spread to, and he answered truthfully and told me it could spread to the lungs and/or bones.

When the surgeon left, Phil and I looked at each other, dazed. I did not know what to say to my husband of nearly 25 years. I felt angry and sad at the same time. I did not want anybody feeling sorry for me, and I imagined Phil now being stuck with an invalid unable to work and a drain on the family finances. Phil being typically male did not show any reaction at all, looked on the bright side, and mentioned again the high survival rate and how it could be cured with the RAI. I knew though that he was trying to be cheerful and not show me how devastated he was. We could not believe this was happening; it was everyone's worst nightmare come true.

I lay back on the pillows and tried to sleep, but the anaesthetic's after-effects ensured I would be wide awake for the next three days. When I did eventually doze off I woke up immediately feeling sick and dizzy each time, and this effect lasted for nearly two weeks after surgery. The amount of phlegm on my chest was bothering me, as I felt I was choking trying to cough it up. When the hostess arrived with the supper for that first evening which I had ordered earlier in the day, I could not eat. I sipped water for the first day and night.

I decided to have a quick look at my medical notes after supper, when the room was empty. I glanced at the front page, and the surgeon had written *'I strongly suspect a neoplasm.'* I resolved to look that word up when I returned home.

CHAPTER 8 - SECOND DAY AFTER SURGERY

On the second day, a nurse suggested I try and get out of bed to go to the toilet. This seemed like a monumental undertaking, as I felt so weak. I could not ever envisage being able to get in and out of the bath again either, but the nurse said not to try that for a few days yet. Phil was on hand to help as I duly swivelled my legs around out of the bed and shakily stood up. My heart immediately started pounding again with the effort. I shuffled the few yards to the toilet and whilst in there made the mistake of looking at myself in the mirror.

My face was a strange brown rusty colour, which I attributed to an allergic reaction to the anaesthetic. The right side of my bottom lip was swollen and sore – goodness knows what had happened to that. An angry looking bright red scar about 3 inches long was present at the bottom of my neck, and below that was a big black bruise on my chest the size of a dinner plate. Horrified, I turned away and after going to the loo got thankfully back into bed. I would not win any beauty contests that day!

The hostess arrived with my porridge and this time I could manage a few mouthfuls with a glass of fruit juice. Things were looking up; I still did not feel sick and I had managed to jettison the bedpans. I was determined to walk to the toilet from now on. I even managed to have a little wash at the sink later in the day.

After breakfast was medicine time. The nurse brought me a fast-acting thyroxine substitute, Liothyronine Sodium (sometimes known as T3). I was to take three tablets per day. The tablets were 20micrograms each, and I would stay on these until two weeks before my RAI treatment when I would need to be off the T3 altogether and on a low iodine diet. As mentioned before this was the only way to make any remaining thyroid cells hungry for iodine and so receptive to the RAI, which would kill them off. If I had been on the proper levothyroxine hormone (sometimes known as T4), I would have had to come off it for six weeks prior to RAI treatment and would have felt very ill indeed (the T4 levels tend to stay constant in the body for longer, whereas T3 is short-acting and only takes two weeks to leave the body). That was the reason I was not given T4 levothyroxine immediately after surgery, as it took about six weeks to leave the body. It only takes about three months without thyroxine for a person to die, so you can imagine how ill you would be after six weeks with no thyroxine at all. It started to sound very complicated and I didn't feel much like trying to get my head around it at that moment. It was to take at least two weeks for the results of the biopsies to come back so I decided I'd worry about it then. It still might not be cancer. I was ever hopeful.

After medicine time and observations came the ward round. The surgeon said I needed to stay another night but could go home the following day. Phil agreed that I would be better off at home, if nothing else it would improve my chances of sleep. I did not actually feel well enough to go home, but went along with everybody else and welcomed the chance to leave hospital – it meant I was well and truly on the road to recovery.

Phil stayed with me for the rest of the day. I tried to doze but sleep eluded me. I was finding it hard to talk. I became out of breath if I tried to say too much all at once. Phil reassured me that because I could only whisper, I had to use more air for talking, which was causing the breathing problem. I was still having trouble coughing, and drinking anything made me splutter and choke. To cap it all I was also getting symptoms of yet another period coming. I could not believe it – one had only finished the week before after 19 days. Exactly the same thing was happening again which had caused me to consult a gynaecologist ten years previously. I would have to go back on the norethisterone tablets. Coupled with the new T4 levothyroxine tablets I would also have to take, I would be rattling. The improved diet was not good enough – I obviously had some major hormone deficiencies!

During the night I got out of bed to go to the toilet but felt very strange as I was walking back to bed. Pins and needles were in my hands and feet and I felt strangely light-headed. It would not go away and I pressed the call button to summon the nurse. She laid me down on the bed, raised my feet a little, and explained I'd had a little 'faint'. She checked my blood pressure, which was quite low. I'd never fainted before so did not recognise the symptoms. She said I had probably got out of bed too quickly, and was to sit on the bed for a few minutes first before getting out next time. I felt like an old lady. I could usually leap out of bed like a scalded cat.

The next day came and I was to go home after lunch. There would be a follow-up appointment two weeks later with the surgeon in his clinic to hear the results of the biopsy. Phil brought the car as near to the back patio doors as he could as I was too weak to walk very far. I still did not feel ready to go home, but said goodbye and thanks to the nurses and doctors, and held Phil's arm as he led me to the car. I sunk into the seat with a grateful sigh – the few yards had seemed like a long trek. We returned home via the GP's surgery. Phil dropped my discharge letter in and collected some more T3 liothyronine sodium tablets to see me through to the RAI treatment a couple of months down the line.

CHAPTER 9 – HOME AGAIN

When I arrived home on the Wednesday, it was early afternoon and Matt was not yet home from work. I could not be bothered to unpack my case and just sat on the sofa figuring out how to tell my son that I probably had cancer. There were also Lee and Sarah to tell who were coming to visit that evening and last but not least my eighty one year old mother who lived nearby. I quickly decided not to tell her, as she was a very anxious person who would doubtless have become very worried at the mention of the word 'cancer', and I could not have handled the dramatics in my delicate state. She would have possibly wrongly assumed I was dying, and would have found it hard to listen to any explanation I would have been able to give. I would tell her my thyroid was removed along with a cyst in order to stop any more cysts growing on it. The surgeon had assured me the survival rate was in the ninety to ninety-five per cent range, so I had high hopes that I wouldn't suddenly deteriorate and shuffle off.

I still felt rather dreadful. I had terrible trouble coughing up the large amount of phlegm that kept accumulating in the back of my throat. My cheeks had lost the rusty brown colour and now had a ghostly grey hue. I was still weak and could not walk far. When Matt was due home, I decided to soften the blow by putting a chiffon scarf around my neck so he could not see the damage done.

Matt bounded in his usual upbeat self and gave me a big hug. I relayed to him the surgeon's probable diagnosis. His face fell, but he also said (as did Phil) that the survival rates were encouraging and of course there might not be any cancer found after the biopsy. He disappeared upstairs to bathe and change and seemed quiet after my revelation, only appearing for dinner and then returning to his room again where quiet acoustic guitar playing could be heard. Matt usually plays loud rock and melodic metal, so something was wrong in his little world. Lee and Sarah popped over for a visit and the same scenario was played out. The look on their faces said it all. Lee went upstairs to talk to Matt for a while.

After Lee and Sarah's short visit, I had another coughing fit and found it difficult to breathe suddenly with the amount of phlegm seemingly in the airway. I told Phil I needed to return to the Nuffield as I did not feel safe at home with no emergency suction, and felt I might drown in my own secretions. Fortunately my bag was still not unpacked. We told Matt that I needed to go back to hospital. By this time it was 9.30 in the evening. Poor Phil felt dreadful as he blamed himself for encouraging me to come home believing it would be in my best interests. He phoned the Nuffield to tell them to expect us back and drove me there all stressed out and upset. I tried not to cough in the car in case I could not breathe in. I hoped no police were around hiding in lay-bys with hand-held mobile speed cameras as we raced back to the Nuffield in record time.

At 10pm we were ringing the night bell. It seemed an eternity before it was answered, as the nurses on duty had been busy tending to patients and could not come down to open the door straight away. I was shown to a different room this time – room 23, which was not as nice as the one I had vacated that afternoon. It was upstairs with obviously no patio doors and garden. As soon as I arrived, I was seen by the admitting nurse who took the usual pulse, temperature, and blood pressure, and then by the in-house doctor who prescribed a course of nebulisers for me to inhale – 4 per day starting that night, to loosen the phlegm. Phil waited until I was settled inhaling the saline nebuliser (the machine was very loud and I'm certain kept the other patients nearby awake) and then went home to bed. I stayed connected to the nebuliser for half an hour or so, and it seemed to help. It was reassuring to be back in the hospital whilst I felt so unwell.

CHAPTER 10 – THREE DAYS AFTER SURGERY AND BEYOND

The next day was three days on from the surgery and I had a visit from the physiotherapist who showed me some breathing exercises to do every half an hour that would give additional help with the phlegm problem. If I had known at the time it would take me about eight weeks to be almost rid of it I would have felt quite depressed! I must have had quite a bad reaction to the anaesthetic, as the phlegm certainly was not there before the operation. On a happier note I could not help but notice that the physiotherapist was a tad on the hunky side (a girl can look can't she?), so I eagerly looked forward to learning further breathing exercises.

There was also a chest x-ray to be done. The surgeon had requested this and Phil and I supposed he wanted to check for any secondary cancers. I was too weak to walk to the X-Ray Department, so a porter came for me pushing a wheelchair. It took all my strength to stand up in front of the x-ray machine. Phil heard the radiographer say to her colleague that she could not see any secondaries, which was encouraging. They told me the x-ray was clear. At least that was one piece of good news. The surgeon also told me on the ward round my chest was clear and that if I felt better the next day, I could go home. The nebulisers were helping to loosen the phlegm, and I felt more able to cope. I agreed to go home the next afternoon.

On the Friday after lunch, we again said our goodbyes. It was a longer walk out of the hospital this time as we had to walk downstairs and then through the reception area and out to the car. I had my little chiffon scarf on again so as not to frighten any unsuspecting out-patients that were waiting in Reception. I chose to walk down the stairs rather than take the lift to prove to myself I could do it. I am terribly stubborn. It took an eternity but I did it clutching onto Phil's arm. I still looked and felt dreadful but somehow knew I would not need to go back yet again.

Back at home I spent the next few weeks recuperating. I still could not move my neck from side to side properly, and to add to my troubles on the second day home, part of the cracked tooth broke off whilst I was eating dinner. Perhaps it had been knocked during the anaesthetising process? I felt like crying into my vegetables – how unlucky can one person get I thought? I felt too weak to manage a visit to the dentist and decided to wait until I felt a bit better. Also during these first weeks my periods returned with such a vengeance that I was getting one every other week and constant PMT symptoms. I gave in and started taking the norethisterone tablets again. At least one problem was solved. Another problem manifested itself though in the vacated space. I suspected the T3 dose of three tablets per day was too high as my heart was constantly pounding, I felt anxious, and was losing weight. I emailed the surgeon who advised me to take two tablets instead, one in the morning and one in the evening, which seemed to agree with me more.

Luckily the weather was warm and I sat in the garden every day not doing much at all. At first Phil had to wash my hair and my back at bath time as the movement pulled on the scar if I tried to do it, but after a couple of weeks I could do this for myself. I trawled the Internet to find out anything I could about my condition. I found thyroid cancer affects mainly middle-aged women and the cause was not known. There are theories that include too much weight gain and sudden weight loss during pregnancy, and radiation to the face or neck during childhood. Even Chernobyl was mentioned. I had had lots of dental x-rays as a child and teenager – perhaps that was the cause? I even toyed with the idea that the norethisterone tablets that I had been taking for 10 years may have caused it, but could not find any evidence to support this. I still could not believe that this had happened to me as I had always taken care of my body. Even now in my weakened state I had started to walk around the village to regain my strength, usually taking the route I used to jog. I love to be outside, and as long as I could still walk, then as far as I was concerned I was okay.

On the 5th July, I attended the Nuffield as an out-patient to see the surgeon and get the results of the biopsy. He confirmed I had papillary thyroid cancer with spread to the surrounding lymph nodes (Stage T4 N1, so quite advanced), as the four swollen lymph nodes that had been removed were also cancerous. He explained papillary cancer was the most common type and easily treatable (the other three types were follicular, medullary, and anaplastic thyroid cancer, with the latter two more difficult to treat successfully). I would have to undergo radioactive iodine (RAI) treatment at Addenbrooke's hospital to kill any remaining thyroid cells (and therefore any cancerous cells), and for this to happen he was going to refer me to a consultant oncologist who worked both at Addenbrooke's and at The Nuffield hospital in Cambridge. Yet another doctor. He was also going to refer me to an ear, nose, and throat (ENT) consultant, to see if he could help with my lack of a voice. It still had not returned a couple of weeks after surgery, and he was getting worried. If he was worried then I was worried, and I wondered if it would ever come back. It was frustrating to try and talk; no voice came out, and people could not hear me. Phil became my voice. I whispered into his ear and he translated to people who could not understand what I was saying.

Over the next few weeks I regained five notes of the scale in the lower register but that was all. There was no power in the voice – if I was talking with one person in a room that was okay – I sounded like an adolescent schoolboy whose voice was breaking. But if I had to talk over background noise and tried to speak louder, nothing came out at all. I actually had to wait until December 2005 to see any real difference in my voice. By then, my speaking voice sounded normal, I had a range of 13 notes, but I still could not shout to get over any background noise (I still can't three years later).

On the 6th July I felt well enough to undergo repairs to the cracked tooth. Phil drove me to our dentist in Long Melford, who gave me a nice white filling. I think he must have felt sorry for me as he charged me the same price as the normal amalgam.

In the second week of July, about a month after the operation I attended Kidbrooke Comprehensive School's reunion of 'old girls'. Looking back, I should have stayed at home as my voice was so weak and the background noise so loud that I could not make myself heard at all. My legs ached from following my friends around all the school corridors where I had run and skipped some thirty years before. With hindsight I realised the T3 levels were falling in the afternoon when I was doing lots of walking around the school (T4 does not cause the same symptoms as levels stay constant in the blood), and I was exhausted when Phil came to collect me in the car and slept most of the way home.

The following day we were scheduled for a week away in the Isle of Wight (renting the bungalow again from Dave's sister) - this time just the two of us. Matt and Anna were off for a week's holiday in Italy, and Lee and Sarah stayed near the hospital as their baby was due the following week. It was a lovely week away from hospitals and doctors. Just before we left for the Isle of Wight a letter arrived from the oncologist with an appointment date to see her at the Nuffield hospital at Cambridge, which I noticed was the very next day after we were due home. I resolved to enjoy my holiday – the first holiday Phil and I had taken alone in over 23 years. We had always taken the boys with us on holiday and now they were grown up we finally had some time to ourselves. We could visit all those National Trust houses instead of children's playgrounds and arcades!

The weather was glorious as we left for the ferry and the sun did not stop shining all week. We lazed on the beach at Puckpool, visited Osborne House and Arreton Manor, sunbathed in the secluded garden of the bungalow, and had a lovely dinner out every night near to the bungalow at The Windmill Hotel in Bembridge. Mary and Dave had been there the previous week and we met up on our first day for lunch before they went home. Only one cloud marred the horizon – the Thursday afternoon of that week saw me sitting in the Accident and Emergency department of the Isle of Wight's main hospital at Newport. My scar was sore and two places were infected and oozing pus. I was not sure what to do with it but the doctor there said it was best to do nothing and leave it alone. He said the two infected places were caused by internal sutures sticking out of the scar. Eventually the stitches would drop out but it might take some time. When I got back to the bungalow I wiped the scar with salt water, which helped with the oozing but it still felt a bit sore.

There was a lovely end to the holiday on the Sunday morning when Lee phoned to tell us we swere grandparents. Little Sophie Emily had been born by emergency caesarean the previous evening on July 16th 2005, and both mother and baby were doing well. We could not wait to catch the ferry back to see her. Although we were not due to get on the ferry until midday, we caught the 9.30am ferry and by 2.30 pm were sitting outside the maternity ward waiting to see our new granddaughter, who of course was absolutely gorgeous.

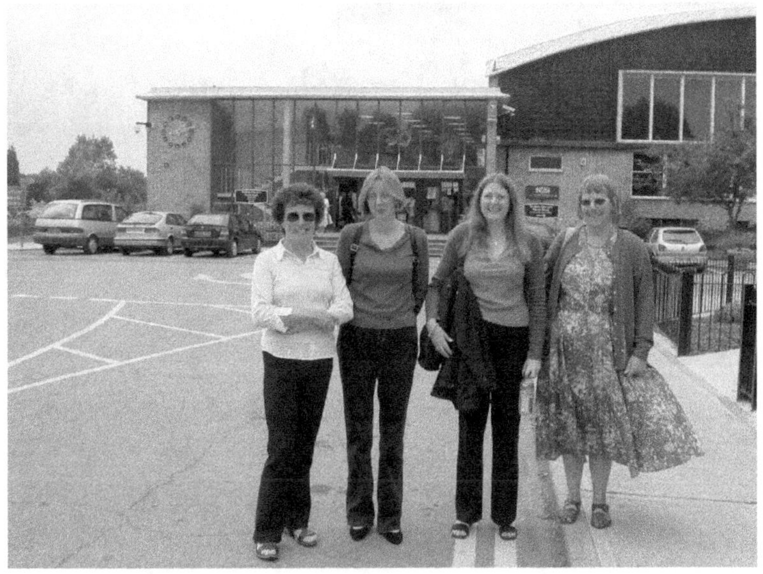

Myself (above left) with some old schoolfriends at
Kidbrooke School reunion, July 2005.

My little granddaughter Sophie at one day old July 17th 2005. Note the scar on my neck from the recent thyroidectomy one month earlier.

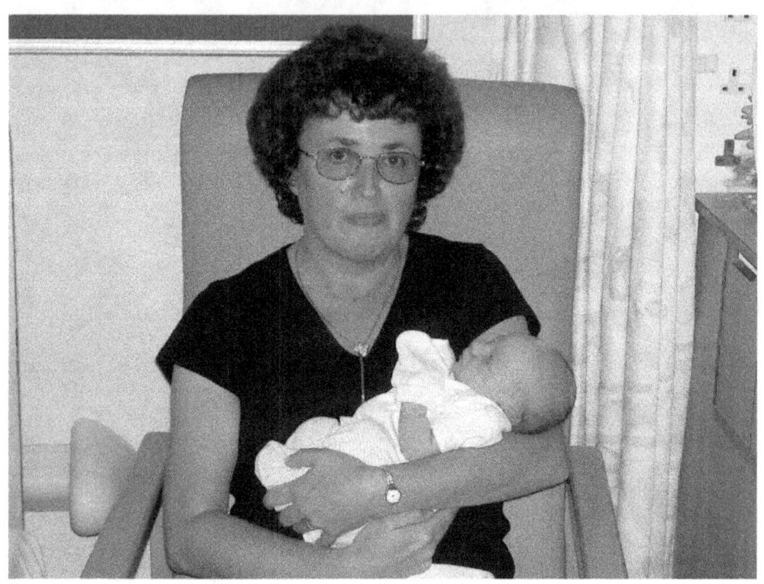

CHAPTER 11 – THE FIRST RADIOACTIVE IODINE TREATMENT

Back to earth with a bump the next day back from holiday. Phil drove me to the Nuffield at Cambridge to meet a new doctor on my ever-growing doctors' Christmas card list. This time I would see a consultant oncologist. She felt my neck and asked how much I had been told of my condition. I filled her in with everything the surgeon had told me and she nodded in agreement. She said she would book me into the RadioIodine Suite at Addenbrooke's as soon as possible and I would have to come off my T3 (liothyronine) tablets for two weeks beforehand in order for the RAI treatment to be effective. This I did not fancy much as I knew I'd feel weak and tired, but it had to be done. I would also have to be on a low iodine diet to make any remaining thyroid cells hungry for the iodine, so no fish or dairy products, and no food with red colouring in it. I did not eat dairy products anyway due to migraines, but it would be hard giving up fish. I would also have to wait for the keyhole surgery to repair my jaw, as she wanted the RAI treatment over with first. That meant taking even more time off work I thought, as now instead of September which I had planned, I would have to wait until probably the summer of 2006 for the locking jaw to be re-aligned.

The oncologist asked me if I wanted to stay a private patient or go through the NHS as the treatment was the same (apart from being treated sooner privately). I wanted it over with soon so told her I would remain a private patient. She said she would phone with the date of the RAI treatment later that day, and she gave me a compliment slip with all her contact numbers on and email address just in case I thought of any questions I wanted to ask her. I did indeed think of many questions over the next fortnight, and she always answered my emails; a very nice lady.

True to her word, she phoned that evening to give me the date of August 8th to go to Addenbrooke's for the start of the treatment. I would have to come off my T3 tablets the following Monday on 25th July. I immediately phoned our local restaurant/pub and booked a table for Sunday lunch – the last day when I could eat normally for a while. Lee and Sarah agreed to come to the lunch and bring baby Sophie along in her pushchair. I did not know how long it would take to start feeling unwell, so I wanted to make the most of it. Dear little Sophie did not murmur throughout the meal at all, and we all enjoyed the afternoon.

In fact during the first week off the T3, I did not feel too bad at all. I could still cut the grass on the Tuesday and take my mother shopping to Sainsbury's on the Friday. I thought the whole procedure seemed like a doddle. However, the second week was quite different. I started feeling quite weary by the second Monday and was unable to do much at all. I had pains in my calf muscles when I tried to walk (muscles cannot contract properly without thyroxine), and so developed a shuffling gait. I laid about on the sofa and wished it was all over. My eyes felt as though they had lead weights on the lids trying to hold them down. Phil had to help with the shopping on the second Friday as my legs refused to move much at all. I slept quite a bit during the day and because my sleep pattern was disrupted, had trouble sleeping properly at night. I looked and felt terrible. By the end of the fortnight my face was pale and puffy and I had put on half a stone in weight despite having a decreased appetite.

On the 8th August I dragged my poor suffering body through the revolving door of Addenbrooke's hospital. The admission letter had said arrive at the RAI Suite on Ward A5 at 10am. Due to my over-eagerness to get there and start on the treatment we arrived an hour early. Because of the painful calf muscles I wanted to keep walking to a minimum, so I waited in the café by the entrance whilst Phil set about locating the ward. He returned after about 10 minutes having found it and spoken to one of the nurses there who informed him we were too early and to come back at 10am! We stayed in the café reading the newspaper.

At 10am we went to the ward and were shown to the purpose-built Radioiodine Suite. At first I was a little disappointed as my room was quite small (one of two leading from a small lobby), and I would be holed up there all week. But at least it had windows which I could look out of (I thought it would be a lead-lined cell!), although there wasn't much of a view. The room also had a free telephone, a television, and my own sink and toilet. The shower room was just outside the door in the lobby. There was a kettle to make myself a hot drink and a toaster. I felt pleased with myself for having remembered to bring herbal tea bags.

A doctor came to take a blood test to check my haemoglobin, thyroglobulin (all thyroid cells produce thyroglobulin, so a high thyroglobulin level above 2 gives an indication that thyroid or thyroid cancer cells are still present), and TSH (thyroid stimulating hormone – which would be high as it had not been suppressed with T3 for a fortnight) levels. He explained that I would be given an anti-sickness pill about half an hour before the RAI drink. This would ensure it stayed down for the two or three hours it would take for my body to absorb it. After that I would need to be isolated and drink a lot of water and take frequent showers to flush it out of my system. He also tidied up the sutures which were still sticking out of the scar. A nurse came in with admission paperwork which I helped her to fill in, and afterwards she gave me an identity wristband to wear. I asked when I could begin to take my T3 tablets again, and was told probably after my scan on Friday (three weeks off T3 is no joke).

The physicist who would administer the drink arrived, checked my identity, and more or less repeated what the doctor had said; I could not go home unless radioactive levels were safe for me to be let out into the community. When he left I looked at Phil and sighed. At last things were underway. I was due to fight my own little war alone in this room against an unseen enemy.

I was then visited by Ann who had worked on the RAI Unit for 16 years. Ever cheerful, it was her job to bring me my meals. She explained that when I was radioactive, she would knock at the door and if I left my table near to the door and sat as far away from the door as possible, she would leave my meals on the table. I would then wash up my plate and cutlery and leave them outside the room for her to collect at a later date when all the rooms had been decontaminated. She brought me a nice lamb stew at midday and some extra pillows and towels. She even said if I gave her the correct change before my RAI drink, she would buy a newspaper for me every day. What a star! If I had left the ward highly radioactive to go down to the shop, I would have set off a loud alarm bell just outside the RAI suite!

After lunch, Phil and I sat about and waited for the RAI drink. At 1.30 I was given an anti-emetic and at 3pm the physicist returned with the drink, which was Phil's cue to leave. He would not be able to visit again until the next day when radioactive levels had dropped somewhat, and then only for 20 minutes each day. He had to enter the room wearing plastic overshoes and gloves and sit as far away from me as possible.

The physicist had a rather large bottle in his hand and my face fell at the thought of having to drink the whole contents – no wonder they gave the anti-emetic first! He laughed and said no; the bottle contained a liquid that I was to sprinkle down the toilet before flushing it which would help to break up the RAI. The drink itself came in a lead-lined box and was only a tiny amount. He checked my identity again with the nurse present, and then inserted 2 needles into the top of the RAI phial. These were attached to 2 plastic tubes, one of which I would drink through like a straw. The end of the other one he put into a cup of water which helped to flush the last of the RAI out of the phial and into me, ensuring I had all of it.

I duly drank the RAI after putting on a plastic apron to guard against splashes, and that was that. The physicist left after taking the first readings. Apparently levels would need to be one quarter of the present reading before I could go home. I resolved to wait half an hour to let the RAI go down before I started drinking. After that, I drank as much water as I felt able to for the rest of the day. Tea consisted of soup and sandwiches, which were put outside my door at 5pm after a call from the reception desk asking if I wanted them. I spent the evening reading, filling in crossword puzzles, and watching television. I made use of the free phone to call Phil, Matthew, and my mother.

The night passed uneventfully as far as feeling nauseous was concerned. I tossed and turned though as air-conditioning units outside droned constantly and the fridge hummed and buzzed inside. At 7am I phoned the desk to make sure I had enough time to take a shower before breakfast. Staff seemed quite helpful and I was assured

Ann would leave my breakfast until last, giving me enough time to wash. After that it was time to occupy myself until the oncologist did her ward round and the physicist returned to check if my radiation levels had decreased.

After lunch consisting of sausages, mash, and vegetables, the oncologist popped her head round the door. She said as soon as the physicist said radiation levels were okay, then I could go home and then come back Friday for a body scan. I could start back taking my T3 tablets the next day, Wednesday. Awesome! I could not wait to be able to walk properly and feel normal again instead of exhausted all the time. I had found out through an Internet support group, that there were thyrogen injections I could have had to stimulate my TSH levels without coming off the T3 tablets. The oncologist's colleague had said the NHS would not fund the injections as they were £250 each, but my medical insurance company would probably pay for them. I made a mental note to ask the oncologist about them during my next follow-up appointment with her at the Nuffield, Cambridge, on September 12th to get my blood test findings and scan results. I would also probably need a second increased dose of RAI in six months' time to ensure all cancer cells had been killed off.

On that second day, the Nurses kept asking if I needed anti-sickness pills as though they were all waiting for me to throw up. I felt I was disappointing them munching my way through all meals put in front of me!

The physicist arrived about 2.30 to check radiation levels. He nodded encouragingly and said levels were a third below the previous day's readings and all being well I could go home the next day. I nearly jumped for joy as it was only a small room and I was getting a touch of cabin fever. I much prefer being outside, so it had been hell.

Phil arrived at 6.15pm for his allotted 20 minutes. He wanted to stay longer but was not allowed. The poor chap was sweating in his rubber gloves and plastic overshoes.

As soon as I woke up on the Wednesday, down the little red lane went the first T3 tablet for nearly 3 weeks. I had to take T3's for one week, and then the proper T4 levothyroxine tablets from then on which would keep my TSH suppressed and hopefully stop any more thyroid/thyroid cancer cells from growing. I noticed my salivary glands were starting to feel a little sore and my mouth was dry so I sucked on some boiled sweets which I had been advised to bring, as they would help by stimulating the salivary glands. The trouble was I was not too keen on boiled sweets (not having much of a sweet tooth), and so could only manage a couple. Lunch was a nice chicken and leek pie with vegetables and then mixed fruit afterwards.

The oncologist visited as usual at 2pm and confirmed I could eat normally when I returned home – no more low iodine diet! I also would not need a certificate of radiation given when we embarked on our cruise in November. I was worried I might have set off airport alarms but she felt sure this would not happen.

At 2.30 the physicist made his usual rounds. He said radioactive levels were low enough for me to go home. He checked all my belongings and said only the clothes I had been wearing were slightly radioactive, but if I washed them separately when I got home and then run the washing machine again empty, that would solve the problem. I could not prepare any food that evening, I was to stay away from public places for the rest of the day, and pregnant women and children for another 3 days. After that I would be back to normal. I was to return for the scan on Friday and could collect my new 200mcg T4 thyroxine tablets from the ward then which would see me through for the next month. I would then need to order them on a repeat prescription from the GP. Luckily I had also found out on the support group that by having a chronic long-term medical condition needing levothyroxine tablets, I would be exempt from prescription charges for life. There is an advantage to having thyroid cancer! Phil arrived at 5.30 to take me home. It was lovely walking out into the fresh air. I'd only had to stay in for 3 days so all in all the first RAI dose had not been as bad as I'd first thought.

CHAPTER 12 – RESULT OF TREATMENT AND 1ST GAMMA SCAN

Funnily enough it was the next day at home when I felt at my worst. My salivary glands felt swollen and sore, I felt sick after dinner, and I still had aching legs and exhaustion from the lack of T3 tablets. I knew it would take quite a few days for the T3 to kick back in, but I sobbed as I wanted to feel better NOW!

On the Friday it was time to return to Addenbrooke's for a Gamma scan. Phil noticed I was walking better along the hospital corridors. Thinking about it, yes, my calf muscles were not as painful; the T3 was starting to work at last. I was still tired, but there was a definite improvement from the day before.

At the Nuclear Medicine department before my scan, the technician asked me to empty my bladder, drink a cup of water to wash any radioactivity from the salivary glands, and remove any metal objects before getting me to climb onto the scanner bed. There were large camera plates above and below me. The technician told me the plates would come quite close to my face but would not actually touch me, and would take pictures from my head to just below my pelvis. I felt rather apprehensive as I suffer from mild claustrophobia and my heart started racing. The technician reassured me she would be in the room with me at all times.

I decided to shut my eyes when the bed moved inside the camera plates so that I would not feel shut-in (I still do this today with any follow up MRI scans), and try to project my mind away from it all. The plates seemed to stay close by my head for ages before I could see more light behind my eyes and sensed they had moved downwards. I opened my eyes and relaxed somewhat after that as my head was outside the scanner. The scan took about 30 minutes and I had to lie as still as possible. No results could be seen straight away. Unfortunately I would have to wait for one month.

1st scan pictures below taken on 12th August 2005 show uptake of RAI in the thyroid bed. There is always uptake in the salivary glands and bladder, so these are discounted.

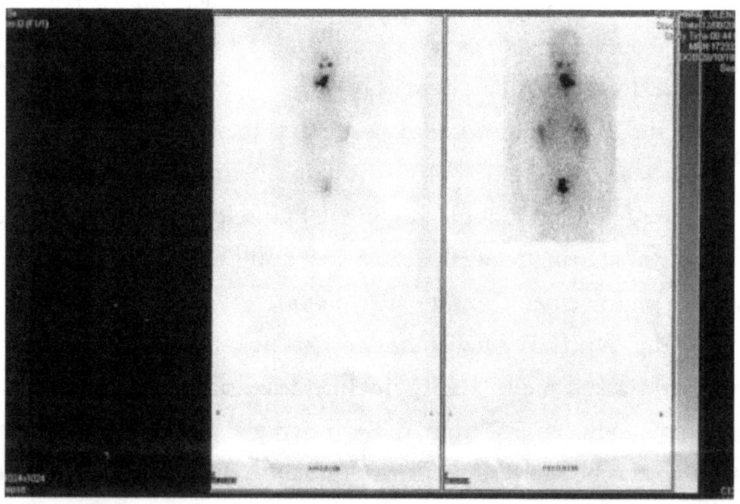

On the first Sunday after my treatment it was wonderful walking along Great Yarmouth seafront. Although the usual East wind was blowing and there was rain in the air, it was a positive tonic after being shut in earlier in the week in the little room on Ward A5. Phil and I sat and froze on the beach and loved every minute of it (well, I did anyway).

When the following Wednesday came around, I could start on the new T4 levothyroxine tablets that I would have to take for the rest of my life. The nursing staff on Ward A5 had said to take them with food as they could be 'rough on the stomach'. The instructions on the packet and the Internet support group for thyroid cancer sufferers said to take them first thing in the morning without food. My GP said it did not matter one way or the other. I was totally unsure what to do, and emailed the oncologist. Back came the answer that it was best to take them on an empty stomach first thing in the morning.

The only drawback I can see from having cancer, is that if any other medical condition presents itself, one immediately thinks the cancer must be returning. Since May I had had a round spot in my vision in my right eye and a couple of weeks after my stay at Addenbrooke's, I was back at my local hospital's Eye Clinic as an NHS patient. I think I am destined never to go too long without a hospital visit. The appointment had been put off since just before my thyroidectomy, and as I sat waiting to see the doctor, I wondered if the cancer had spread to my eye. I told myself not to be so stupid and to wait and see what the doctor would say.

I was told there was a leaky blood vessel on my retina which was causing the spot, it was nothing to do with the cancer – it was just one of those things that happen sometimes. It looked to be resolving itself though, but just to be on the safe side, I would have to come back in a few weeks' time and have an injection of an iodine based dye so that the medical photographer could take some pictures and see if the blood vessel was still leaking. If it was, it could be zapped with a laser. I thought I'd better check with the oncologist to see if this procedure (called a Fluorescein Angiography) would be ok for me to undergo, as I would be pumped with iodine again.

I got to see her again at her monthly Thyroid Clinic at Addenbrooke's. Although I had an appointment to see her on 12th September at Cambridge's Nuffield hospital, another appointment had come through the post for 6th September for the NHS Thyroid Clinic at Addenbrooke's, which had probably been automatically generated by the staff on Ward A5. Phil and I duly made our way to the clinic on the 6th September. I was nervous, as I knew I would probably get the result of the scan and was worried that the cancer had spread. I imagined chemotherapy, losing my hair, having to cancel our 25th anniversary cruise booked for 18th November – my imagination was running riot and my heart was beating fast ('catastrophising' I think they call it!)

My heart sank when I saw the queue of people sitting in Clinic 12's waiting area on that Tuesday morning. Everybody had scars on their necks though, so I felt right at home. As Phil and I were looking round for a seat, the oncologist walked past and asked what we were doing there, as she had not expected to see me until the following Monday at the Nuffield. That was a good start.

Fortunately I was called right on time. I sat down in the consulting room next to Phil and thought my heart would burst out of my chest as it was pounding so much. I had nothing to fear. The oncologist explained that the uptake of the radioiodine had all been in my neck area only, so the cancer had not spread (as far as she could tell). I breathed a sigh of relief. I would need another dose of RAI the week beginning January 16th 2006 as my thyroglobulin level was above normal and the scan showed uptake in the neck area, but in the meantime could go on my cruise, have holiday vaccinations, and have my iodine dye injected in my local hospital's Eye Clinic.

I was told to forget about doctors and hospitals until January; I just needed a blood test so that she could check if I had enough thyroxine in my system to keep the thyroid stimulating hormone suppressed. I was also told that I could have thyrogen injections before my second RAI treatment, so that I would not need to come off the T4 tablets (apparently with the first RAI dose it is advisable to always come off the T3 tablets and have thyrogen injections on subsequent treatments).

I nearly floated out of the consulting room and did not even mind the long wait in Addenbrooke's blood testing area. Phil seemed even more relieved than I was, and we hurriedly posted off the outstanding balance for the cruise on the way home (I had kept the money back in case we had to cancel due to my ill-health, chemotherapy etc.). At Addenbrooke's I had seen a fellow sufferer from the Internet support group who was also waiting for a blood test. She had undergone not only a thyroidectomy, but two neck dissections as well due to spread to the lymph nodes. Her neck looked like a map of the Norfolk broads. I thanked my lucky stars I only had one small scar.

The week following the visit to the Thyroid Clinic was nearly six weeks after my first dose of radioactive iodine. It had taken all this time for the T4 levothyroxine levels to come up, and I was noticing that my heart was pounding at a very fast rate even when I was sitting still, and that my body was giving off so much heat that my glasses were steaming up on the inside! I had a nasty feeling the dose was too high, so I emailed the oncologist and waited for her reply. She emailed back saying the results of the blood test at the Thyroid Clinic showed that the thyroxine dose of 200mcg was too high and that I was to reduce to 175mcg per day. That was fair enough, but I only had 100mcg tablets. Yet another visit to the GP surgery ensued to get some 50mcg and 25mcg tablets, as the 100mcg tablets were too small to cut up accurately. Now I would have to wait for another six weeks for the new dose to stabilise, and then have another blood test to check the level. Having thyroid cancer treatment seemed a very long-drawn out process I was beginning to realise!

On the 21st September I faced yet another doctor but this time back at the Nuffield at Bury St Edmunds. This time it was the consultant ENT surgeon, and I was hoping there would be something he could do for my weak voice. I still only had a few tones in the lower register after three months, and a kind of two-tone breathy whisper in the upper regions. Singing was out of the question, which was making me quite depressed, as I am a very musical person and to sing along to a song was second nature to me.

The ENT surgeon gave me a local anaesthetic through my nose which numbed the back of my throat (fortunately) and he then began threading a camera on the end of a long tube through my nose down the back of my throat so that he could see the vocal cords. The experience was most disagreeable, and I had to use the 'shut my eyes and project my mind away from it all' strategy. He asked me to count to ten. He could see as I was talking that my left vocal cord was paralysed and that the right one was trying to compensate, but to not much effect. The nerve had either been severed or damaged through manipulation during the operation. The endocrine surgeon had told him he had had trouble in removing my lymph glands, so the manipulation had probably caused the damage. The ENT surgeon suggested leaving well alone for at least six months to see if the vocal cord improved, as in his experience there was often improvement six to nine months later, and he didn't want to operate and then find afterwards the vocal cord had healed by itself, thus negating any surgical repair work which had been carried out too early.

I left the Nuffield after making an appointment to see him again in March 2006, which would be the day after my appointment with the maxillo-facial oral Surgeon, who would hopefully give me a date to re-align my jaw. If an operation on my vocal cords was necessary, I wanted both operations to be carried out at the same time so that I would only have to recover from one anaesthetic. On mentioning this to the ENT surgeon, he could see no problem with this and even said the oral surgeon's presence would probably be necessary anyway as my jaw would have to be opened as wide as possible to access the vocal cords (I was rather relieved that my scar would not be re-opened). Deep joy.

CHAPTER 13 – NEW JOB & VISIT TO THE EYE CLINIC

Meanwhile my workplace managers were starting to wonder when I would be returning to work. My ward manager had envisioned I would need only three weeks off work initially to recover, but this had stretched to nearly four months as although I felt recovered, my voice was so weak I knew I would not be able to answer the phone which rang constantly on the ward, or be able to do much talking to ward visitors. I had frittered away the whole summer sitting outside on my favourite piece of garden furniture, the 'Timewaster' (a kind of swinging chair with a canopy).

The Clinical Manager suggested a meeting on September 22nd which I duly attended. After I had told her my problems with speaking for any length of time, she suggested re-deployment and asked me if I would be interested in a secretarial assistant vacancy in the Cardiology Department, as she had had only good reports regarding my work and she wanted to give me a chance to work again. The job would mostly involve typing letters and reports.

I could not believe my luck. Not only was a secretarial assistant a grade 3 post (my current post was grade 2) so there would be a higher salary, it was the sort of job I had been after for some time but somebody else always beat me to it. This time I would face no competition – the job was mine! I was to start work on 3rd October.

I positively skipped back to the car – I had begun to think that due to my illness I would be on the scrapheap regarding work and job prospects. How wrong I was! I would be on a three months trial and I vowed to work as hard as I could to show them how well I could do the job. There would be times when I would have to take time off to have treatment in the Eye Clinic and to undergo radioactive iodine therapy at Addenbrooke's, so I hoped that people didn't feel sorry for me and think I was totally unhealthy and a lost cause.

I spent the next week excitedly shopping for new work clothes and spending a great deal of my September's salary in the process. October 3rd arrived, and feeling very nervous I reported as asked to the manager who was in charge of all the secretaries. She took me along to my new office upstairs situated in the corridor of the new Cardiology ward. There were two secretaries there who turned out to be very friendly, helpful, and went out of their way to answer any questions I had, and I had many. There was a whole new specialised vocabulary to learn, names of drugs to learn how to type and audio typing to get to grips with, especially deciphering the heavily accented voices coming at me through the headphones. Within a week I knew I loved the job and wanted to stay there. The other girls helped me as much as they could during that first week including the other two part-time secretaries who only worked a couple of days a week each.

I thought I would feel really tired that first week, but as I was sitting down for most of the day I did not feel too bad – I had felt more tired in my previous job at the end of the day in which I had been much more active. I was beginning to get back to my normal self; the only nagging pains were an occasional pain in my left collar bone and the teeth on the right side of my mouth were sometimes painful, but I had a high pain threshold and decided to live with it. The hardest thing of all was trying to reassure myself that not every pain was the cancer coming back – it was probably the aches and pains of getting older.

I was still feeling hot most of the time though, and suspected the 175mcg Thyroxine was still too high. Blood tests revealed this was so, and I was switched to 150mcg and felt a good deal better on this dose, but still hot sometimes. However I was still over-medicated but the oncologist did not want me to come down any more, as 150mcg was keeping the TSH level suppressed which would hopefully stop any more thyroid cancer tissue from growing, and she thought it dangerous to drop the dose to 125mcg as that was too low. I would have to be over-medicated for the rest of my life. I read that too much thyroxine in the system made you susceptible to osteoporosis, and resolved to ask the oncologist about that when I went to Addenbrooke's in January for my second RAI dose.

October 3rd was also memorable for another reason. Having gone to bed happy at the way my first day back at work had gone, I was woken up by Matthew at 1.30am. He never usually wakes me up. I assumed he was sick but he assured me he was not. He then dropped a bombshell that kept me awake for the rest of the night worrying and fretting. He had found a lump in his testicle whilst showering that evening and the poor boy had been lying in bed obviously worried to death until he just had to tell somebody. I told him that he needed to be seen by the GP as soon as possible to get it investigated, and he agreed. I took pains to tell him just because he had a lump, it didn't mean he had cancer – it could be anything. He went back to bed but neither of us slept – I had only just finished Lance Armstrong's autobiography about how he beat testicular cancer and went on to win the Tour de France seven times, and what with my family's medical history, I must admit I feared the worst.

However, a visit to the doctor's surgery the next day reassured all of us. The GP was almost 100% sure it was a twisted vas deferens and made an appointment for Matthew to have a scan to confirm it. My son's face after coming home from the doctor's was a picture of happiness. I only hoped the doctor knew what he was talking about, and that my diagnostic nightmare was not about to be repeated with Matt. We awaited the appointment for the scan. Only the week before I had said to Phil something along the lines of 'I wonder what else God is going to throw at us in 2005'. The appointment for Matt's scan arrived and was scheduled for October 24th. Thankfully all was well and was just as the doctor had diagnosed.

I had only been at my new job for 3 weeks when it was time to take another day off for my Fluorescein Angiograph of my eye on October 20th. First of all the nurses tested my vision by getting me to read the letter chart. This I managed with flying colours – so far so good. Then it was time to have some local anaesthetic drops put in my eyes and drops to dilate my pupils so that the technician could take the photos of the back of my eye. A cannula was put in my hand for the dye to be injected into, and then I was taken into the photography room. The whole procedure was rather unpleasant, as when the pupils are dilated you are very sensitive to bright lights. As the dye was injected into the cannula, the technician snapped away, but each photo was accompanied by a brilliant flash of light that gave me a headache by the end of it. Being an allergic sort of girl, the nurse was concerned that I might feel sick or faint as the dye was injected, but happy to say I felt okay. When the procedure was over and I stepped outside the room, everything looked alarmingly pink but thankfully that wore off after about 10 minutes.

I sat down with Phil to recover for 10 minutes or so, and he said I looked as though I should be auditioning for 'The Simpsons' as not only did I sound like Marge Simpson due to the paralysed vocal cord, I now looked like her as my skin was tinged yellow! What a prince. He has a warped sense of humour! When I was called back in to get the results of the photos, the doctor said it was an inactive change to the retinal layer which would resolve itself. There was nothing to be done other than to keep a check on it. I would have to live with the black spot in my vision. I would need a follow-up appointment three months hence, which I made for 26th January 2006. We went home where I drank as much as I could to flush the yellow dye out. My urine was bright yellow for a couple of days and I took the following day off work so that people didn't think I had hepatitis A or cirrhosis of the liver. Another medical problem resolved. Two down and just the voice and the jaw to go – that's if something else didn't appear in the meantime…

CHAPTER 14 – HAPPIER TIMES

Yet more time was to be taken off work from November 18th to December 5th, but this time for a much happier reason. Phil and I finally had the dream holiday that we had promised ourselves years back when the boys were growing up and we had spent countless holidays in children's playgrounds. We really pushed the boat out so to speak and went on a P&O cruise to the Caribbean on their newest cruise ship 'Arcadia'. It was really to celebrate our 25th wedding anniversary which had fallen on October 11th, but I suppose we were also celebrating my new lease of life.

We had a wonderful time visiting Barbados, Grenada, Dominica, Tortola, Catalina Island, Grand Cayman, Costa Maya, Cozumel, and Fort Lauderdale in the good old USA. The ship was a massive floating paradise catering to our every whim, and the Goanese crew did everything they could to make our holiday special. The temperature averaged 82°F every day and Christmas seemed a long way away when you were sitting on a Caribbean beach (back home it was snowing with ho-ho-hoing Santas appearing in every shop window)! We flew home from Miami airport on 3rd December to temperatures somewhat lower!

Two other happy events presented themselves in December. I was told my three- month trial at work was up and that I could keep my new job. It was on a fixed-term basis, but my manager had every faith that my contract would be renewed each year. She even said she was pushing for it to be a grade higher (more money!). Also I was aware that six months after the thyroidectomy, my voice had suddenly become much better. Up until the end of October I had only a five maybe six note range, but a month or so later I could sing one octave plus two more notes – 12 notes in all; the relief ! I could sing along to all my CD's in my car on the way to work. I noticed I had to take more breaths than before when I tried to sing though, and could not manage to sing a fast song all the way through, as I would be gasping for breath, but could just about manage if it was a slow song though.

Maybe the consultant ENT surgeon would not need to repair my vocal cord after all? He had referred me to an NHS speech therapist and when I came back from holiday there was a letter telling me I was now on the waiting list. What with my body slowly repairing itself and speech therapy, maybe there would be one operation cancelled and only one more to go (the jaw)? I would still go along to my appointment with the ENT surgeon in March, but was starting to think that maybe nothing would need to be done. It would be a good Christmas this year for me. Not so for poor old Rick Parfitt from one of my favourite rock bands Status Quo, who had to cancel the rest of Quo's UK tour as a growth had been found on his larynx. He was due to have exploratory surgery the week before we were to attend a Quo concert on 17th December at Wembley. Poor old Rick would probably never sing again as they already suspected cancer. It had worked out all right so far for me, but I had my doubts about Rick. I had no need to worry; Rick was soon to be back rocking, as the nodes were benign. He could enjoy his Christmas with his family. His voice was never the same afterwards though, but good for him to not give up touring and singing with the band. He was going to rock 'till he dropped (my sentiments exactly).

Christmas arrived with its usual flurry of visiting relatives, and relatives to be visited. Christmas Day lunch was spent at the Punch and Judy pub in Cardinal Park, Ipswich, with Lee, Sarah, Sophie (good as gold all day – never murmured!) Matt, Anna, and my mother. Boxing Day was spent at Phil's parents' house in Hastings, and there was a New Year's Eve dance and buffet at the Riverside Club in Stowmarket with Matt, Anna, Anna's parents and a couple of their friends. It was the perfect Christmas that was spoilt by only one thing. Over the Christmas holidays I had found a dark round lump inside my mouth on my right inner cheek. I did not tell a soul all over Christmas, especially Phil, as I did not want to spoil anyone's fun. I did tell him when the holidays were over, but nobody else knew. His face gave away no indication as to his thoughts. I was hoping the lump might have gone away during the holidays, but it had not. I wondered hopefully if the lump was due to my sometimes accidentally biting the inside of my mouth due to my jaw being out of alignment (I often woke in pain due to biting my cheek inadvertently whilst asleep).

Finally I knew what I had to do. At the beginning of January I emailed my oncologist and she quickly replied that she had got me an appointment with a colleague of hers at the maxillo-facial clinic at Addenbrooke's on the morning of 16th January when I was due to go in anyway for my second dose of radioactive iodine. Hey ho - another doctor! I was beginning to fear I had another type of cancer. I had only just drawn a line under 2005 and now cancer was rearing its ugly head again. The thought that I might have the big C a second time dominated my thoughts during the early days of 2006.

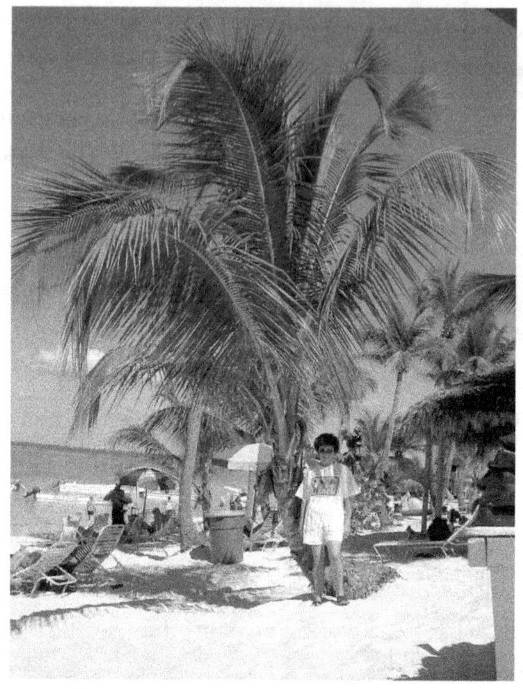

Photo above shows myself on Catalina Island in the Caribbean, November 2005.

CHAPTER 15 – SECOND RADIOACTIVE IODINE TREATMENT

Monday January 16th came round far too soon and Phil and I started off early for my week's stay in Addenbrooke's for the second radioactive iodine dose and to attend the Maxillo-Facial Clinic. This time the district nurse had visited me during the previous two days to administer two doses of thyrogen (total cost £500 thankfully paid by medical insurance) by intramuscular injection. This at least spared me the listlessness, weight gain, pain on walking etc. that had dogged me the last time when I had to come off the T3 tablets. The oncologist said it was necessary only for the first dose of radioactive iodine to stop taking T3. Thankfully this time I had carried on as normal and gone to work. If I had had to stop taking my thyroxine tablets I would not have been able to work after a few days and yet more time would have had to be taken off. The thyrogen injections made any remaining thyroid cells receptive to the radioactive iodine. Coming off of thyroxine would have done the same job also, but I would have felt tired as before and not be able to walk properly.

Thankfully I suffered no ill-effects from the injections, despite the long list of side-effects contained in the blurb that came with the thyrogen powder. After the first injection (embarrassing because the injection was in my behind and administered by a district nurse who had worked on my ward when I was a ward clerk) I sat there and waited to throw up, faint, run to the loo, or goodness knows what else, but nothing happened at all.

We firstly visited the Maxillo-Facial Outpatients' Clinic where I was to be seen by the Addenbrooke's oral surgeon, but unfortunately the reception staff there knew nothing about me. Enquires were made to Ward A5 where I would once again be staying on the Iodine Suite, and surprisingly he was waiting for me there in my little room. Back we trooped to Ward A5 to be told by the oral surgeon that the lump was nothing to worry about, it was self-inflicted due to me biting the inside of my mouth whilst asleep. Well; that was a weight off my shoulders! It had been troubling me all over Christmas in case it had been a secondary.

The routine seemed unchanged from the first time I stayed on the ward. Cheery Ann was still there giving out meals. I was given the other room this time, so at least it was a change from the familiar four walls of the first room. The physicist visited during the afternoon and administered a slightly higher dose of radioactive iodine than before that would hopefully kill off any thyroid cells left. Then it was the usual drinking, showering and sitting about for a couple of days waiting to be told I was no longer emitting radiation and I could leave the room and go home. I was pleased to discover that I was suffering no side-effects this time. The oncologist had told me that the second time around there is less thyroid tissue for the radiation to cling to (it doesn't cling to any other part of the body except the thyroid) and the radiation tends to leave the body quicker. The first time I experienced painful salivary glands, but on the second visit there was nothing.

The boredom was intense though, and the RadioIodine Suite was so hot that I wanted to climb out of the window (it would not open far enough) and feel the cold fresh air on my face (hyperthyroid patients are very intolerant to heat). Because it was winter, the heat was on full blast. I hate heat. The food was terrible – much worse than before. I could only think hospital finances must have been severely strained when only fatty mincemeat and dubious unrecognisable offerings came my way. Thank goodness for Phil bringing in fruit and fruit smoothies made by his own sausage fingers. The dear man had also bought me a portable DVD player for Christmas, so I was able to pass a few pleasant hours watching my favourite films.

I remembered to ask the oncologist about osteoporosis when she visited my room (being over-medicated on thyroxine can cause this). She said there was only a slight risk but she would organise a bone scan in the future, about two years down the line. Funnily enough, an uninvited letter from the Mobile Bone Density Screening Service had arrived in the post the week before, inviting me to pay £35 for a bone ultrasound scan for osteoporosis. My medical records were obviously easily available on computer, and they thought they'd target me I suppose as I was on too much thyroxine. I thought it was a good idea though and made an appointment for Saturday January 21st.

I was allowed to go home, as before, on the Wednesday afternoon (I virtually ran out of the ward and down the stairs, eager to get outside) and was to come back for a scan two days later. The results of the scan and the blood tests taken (to determine thyroglobulin levels which gives an indication if any more thyroid cells are present) would not be available for another two months. I decided to forget about the results for the whole of the intervening time and not worry about it at all, as I would have been a nervous wreck by my appointment date at Cambridge's Nuffield Hospital on Monday March 13th. The scan was easier to tolerate as this time as I was allowed to play my 'Queen with Paul Rodgers' CD, so I kept my eyes shut and concentrated on the music, trying to forget the enormous camera plate was centimetres from my nose. The technicians appreciated the music as they were heartily cheesed off with Addenbrooke's grim choices of Sixties' singalong CD's. I suppose many of the patients were teenagers back in the Sixties, but unfortunately the technicians were not.

Scan on 20th Jan 06 showing RAI uptake in salivary glands and bladder only (usual).

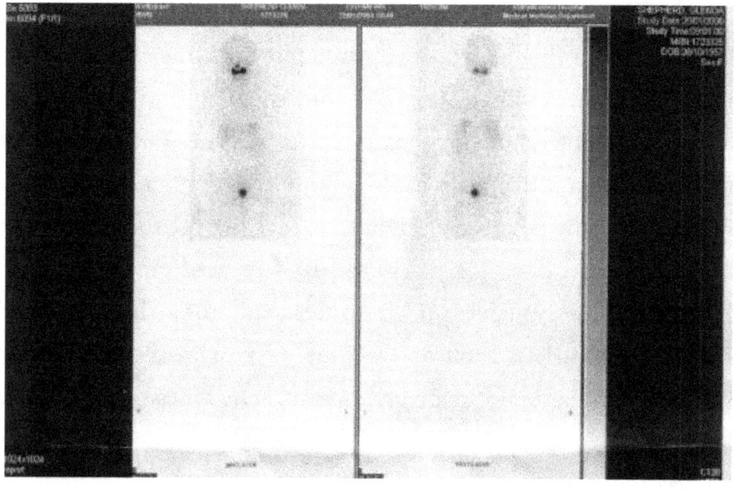

Finally that was it; I could get back to normal and return to work the following Monday. The second dose had been given and hopefully I would be given the all clear in March and not need a third dose.

The following weekend I attended the Mobile Bone Density Screening Unit parked in a local GP surgery car park. All I had to do was take off the sock and shoe from my left foot (as I am right-handed I was told the left side was a little weaker) and place my foot upon the small scanner. The heel was always scanned, as it was the greatest weight-bearing bone. Some acoustic gel was placed on both sides of my foot near the heel, and the scanner then did its thing for a few minutes. The result was so good that the operator decided to do a scan on my right foot as well to check there wasn't a mistake. All that jogging over the previous 10 years had strengthened my bones and on the resultant graph where the central black reference line to aim for was 100%, I was 139%! Some good results for a change! Unfortunately although the jogging does give you strong bones, it does nothing for the joints and I was starting to get achy knees from time to time. I still felt good after a jog though, and had started it up again when my strength returned as I enjoyed it so much. At least I wasn't going to get osteoporosis in the near future. Unfortunately the jogging would end for good in the spring, as my knees started to become painful when I ran. I was still determined I would do some kind of exercise, and from then on began to walk as fast as I could for at least half an hour every day. The knees stopped hurting, and all was well.

CHAPTER 16 – ALL CLEAR?

I could not bear to be away from a hospital for too long (!), so I decided to bring forward my appointment to see the ENT surgeon at Bury's Nuffield hospital. Since the beginning of February my nose had been sore and bleeding from time to time. Phil mentioned going to see the GP about it, but I thought it was not worth it as he would have only referred me to an ENT Consultant and I had been due to see him in March about my voice anyway. I phoned the Nuffield and brought my appointment forward to 15th February. I felt certain he would tell me my vocal cord was working again as I seemed to be speaking normally as long as there wasn't any loud background noise.

The ENT surgeon placed the hated scope in my nostril and down the back of my throat (thankfully he gave me another local anaesthetic that numbed the gagging reflex). He again asked me to count from one to ten. Unfortunately he could see that the vocal cord was still paralysed, but the other one was compensating quite well. He said there was an operation he could do to strengthen it, but as my voice wasn't too bad I would not notice much of a difference. In my nose he could see a raw patch on the septum. He did not think it was to do with my 'other business', but thought it was an infection for which he prescribed some antibiotic cream. I was to return in a month's time so he could look at my nose again. He did not think it was worth doing anything regarding the voice until at least a year had passed since the operation, and it had only been eight months.

Disappointed that my vocal cord was still paralysed and probably always would be, I left the consulting room and made another appointment for 15th March.

Over the next couple of weeks my nose started to feel better and was not so tender. The bleeding stopped and I did not think the ENT surgeon would find anything when he looked a second time.

Meanwhile back at work things were moving on apace. I had only been in my new secretarial job since October, when my manager approached me mid-February to ask whether I would like a Grade 4 medical secretary's post, as I was coping well with Grade 3 work, my current post was only temporary, and she wanted me to be in a permanent post. Since becoming a medical secretary had been my original aim back in 2002 when I joined the NHS, I quickly said yes. I could not believe my luck at the way things were turning out. I only hoped I'd be up to the job, which I knew could be very pressurised, with phones ringing constantly and a constant backlog of work to process. I was able to talk normally on the telephone now, so that was in my favour. I was to work for a world-renowned pain consultant, his associate specialist, a team of clinical nurse specialists, an acupuncturist, and a pain counsellor, along with two other secretaries. I would be typing clinic letters, booking appointments for patients, sorting administration, and answering the telephone etc.

With much trepidation I started work as a medical secretary in the Pain Department on Wednesday February 22nd 2006. For the first few days most of it went straight over my head, but I slowly started getting to grips with it and found I was enjoying it and had found my little niche in life. The much-in-demand pain consultant had thriving private and NHS practices, and gave lectures all over the world on pain relief. It had taken thyroid cancer to get me the job I wanted in the first place! If I had not lost my voice I would probably still have been a ward clerk. The saying 'every cloud has a silver lining' was definitely true for me!

To top it all, the oncologist emailed me at the beginning of March to say that my thyroglobulin (Tg) level had decreased from 4.9 at the first RAI dose down to 1.5 by the second, which was within normal limits (normal being 2 or less). Over time my Tg count would decrease even more to undetectable levels once the TSH was suppressed again. Also my 2nd scan had shown no abnormal uptake, so I could consider myself free from disease! The oncologist still wanted to see me though on 13th March to show me the scan pictures and to inform me of future check-up procedures. The New Year was definitely turning out better than the previous!

The oncologist was all smiles as I met her that morning of the 13th March 2006. She confirmed I was all clear, and would need six-monthly check-ups for the first two years and thereafter yearly check–ups. My first check-up was scheduled for 16th October and I would need a blood test a month before that where TSH and thyroglobulin levels would be checked again. As long as the TSH was kept suppressed with the correct amount of thyroxine and the thyroglobulin level under 2, the cancer would hopefully not return. After a clean scan, if the thyroglobulin level started to rise, it would be assumed that more thyroid cancer cells were growing. I said I was feeling fine on 150mcg of thyroxine without too many side-effects. I only occasionally felt hot, and could hear my heart pounding in my ears only if I bent forward. She decided to keep me on 150mcg for the time being. I could also now go ahead with the jaw operation, and decided to ask the oral surgeon if that could be booked in for July 2006. Hopefully after this I would need no more operations.

I toyed with the idea of finally telling my mother that I had had thyroid cancer but was now all clear, but I decided to go along with the 'ignorance is bliss' theory. That would have worked but after having submitted my story to a press agency, there was a chance it could be published (it wasn't). I had to tell her before the nation read about it. She took it better than I'd expected actually. Because she'd had cancer herself and survived, she understood you don't automatically die just because you've been diagnosed with the disease. She had wondered if it was cancer, but had not liked to ask.

Also, after the usual long wait on the NHS, the speech therapist contacted me in March to ask if I still needed an appointment. As my voice had improved dramatically, I did not think an appointment was necessary, so she said she would send me information in the post of how to look after my voice. I still had the option of surgery in the future, but did not think any speech therapy would make a huge difference.

CHAPTER 17 – EMPTY NEST

I had decided that having cancer was not altogether a negative experience. It had improved my career prospects for a start. It had also made me re-define my priorities in life. I now did not worry about much at all; things in the past that would have caused me sleepless nights now did not bother me. As long as you have your health and a loving family, nothing else matters. I also counted each new day as a bonus because had the 'multinodular goitre' been left untreated, I would most probably not have survived much past my 50th birthday.

Also I realised that doctors are not infallible and can sometimes make misdiagnoses. The radiologist who had given me the ultrasound scan a year before and had diagnosed the 'multinodular goitre' was quite a respected consultant in the hospital where I work, and also one of its directors. His scan report had been sent to the endocrinologist who had probably based his findings on it, and consequently no alarm bells had rung straight away. It was a good thing I had decided myself to have the lump surgically removed, as four years down the line I am still here, but who is to say I would have been if the lump had been left alone?

The only cloud on my now bright horizon was that Matthew announced he would be leaving home to share a rented house with Anna and some of Anna's friends who were all studying music at Homerton College, Cambridge. He would start looking for work local to the college. They were going to view a 5-bedroomed house in Cherry Hinton Road on Saturday March 11th 2006. The last bird was fleeing the nest and I knew I would definitely have the 'Empty Nest Syndrome'. Although Matt was more often out than at home, I always knew he would be returning at some point for his dinner and a chat and I would have to get used to not seeing him so often. His brother had moved out three years previously and I had slowly got used to his absence, but it would be much different with no boys in the house at all. I had nightmare visions of wandering the house looking for my elusive children.

Matt phoned home very excited later on that day. They had decided to take the tenancy of the house, and could move in any time from July 1st onwards. My nightmare would soon be a reality. It's only now when faced with an empty nest that I realise what my own mother, a widow at the time, must have gone through when her only child, me, decided to leave home. My father had died the year previously in 1977, and I had jumped ship aged 20 as soon as I could find somebody to share a flat with. In the long run it helped her though, as she learned to drive, bought a car, took herself dancing and found new friends and even a boyfriend for a while. Perhaps with all this new-found freedom, I would be able to learn to ski, salsa, abseil or whatever - the world was mine for the taking!

It made no difference at first – I pined and pined for my little boy. I gradually came to realise (as does every mother) that I was pining for his lost childhood and because I was not needed any more now that my little boy was a fully grown man. Of course I knew Matt was entitled to a life of his own, but it's not something that a mother can get used to straight away. It took a year or so for me to become used to his absence, and I'm sure Matthew and Anna are very happy that I did. Our children are only loaned to us for a short time, and we must let them go when they are ready.

CHAPTER 18 - SECONDARIES

Fast forward a few months. Matt had settled with Anna in the house in Cherry Hinton Road, Cambridge, and would be joined by the other four students towards the end of September. He had found engineering work in nearby Sawston, and was enjoying the challenge of being given a new type of CNC lathe to work on. There would be promotion for him and a pay rise in 2007 when he had mastered it and its programming complexities. Phil and I (well, Phil was anyway) were slowly getting used to just the two of us in the house, but were still following the band around to gigs. Matt had joined a new band when he left for Cambridge. This band were more focused, more musically competent, and certainly looked as if they might be going places. Lee and Sarah were happy and little Sophie was beginning to crawl about.

I had had an arthroscopy of my left jaw joint done in late July under a general anaesthetic at the Nuffield hospital at Ipswich, but unfortunately I knew the operation had not been a success. In fact the joint was worse than ever, locking during the day, locking whilst eating, locking all night, and making a horrible clicking noise every time I opened my mouth. To top it all, after the arthroscopy I was only allowed to eat pureed food for six weeks to give the joint a chance to heal. The kitchen staff in the hospital at work were very kind and made me a pureed lunch every day, but I could not understand why I was feeling queasy every day about two hours after eating it. On further discussion with the kitchen staff, I found out they were putting fortified milk powder in the soup (I have a really bad milk intolerance) and I was having to pull over to the side of the road on the way home every day because I felt so sick!

The oral surgeon said more invasive surgery was needed that would correct the problem. I needed a meniscectomy – removal of the meniscus disc in the joint. He hadn't wanted to do that first off as he had hoped the keyhole arthroscopy to remove debris and scar tissue would have sufficed. I did not fancy any more anaesthetics and surgery at that time, so decided to put it off until the New Year. A week or so before the arthroscopy I had also had a temporary crown put on the troublesome back tooth that was cracked. It was September before the actual crown could be put on, as the arthroscopy had caused me to be unable to open my mouth properly for six weeks, so the Dentist could not have fitted the permanent crown properly before then. This delay caused an infection in the temporary crown that would not go away.

Also in September it was time for me to get a blood test done, so the results would be ready for my six-month check-up with the oncologist at The Nuffield hospital, Cambridge. I thought I may as well get the blood test done whilst at work, so quickly popped down to Pathology early on 4th September 2006. I knew the thyroglobulin test would take some time to come back, so decided to put the result to the back of my mind for a month or so. I was all-clear anyway, so I assumed the result would be 2 or lower. I actually forgot about checking the result until the day before Phil and I were to leave for a week's holiday at the usual Isle of Wight bungalow at the end of September. No doctor had been in touch with the result. I actually asked a colleague at work to look up the result. It came back 10.2.

The holiday was spoilt for me, as I knew the cancer had come back (had it ever really gone away?). The result should have been 2 or under, and here it was staring me in the face at 10.2 (when the thyroid cancer was first diagnosed, the thyroglobulin had been 78 which had dropped to 4.9 after the first RAI dose). The night before we went away, I hurriedly emailed my oncologist (who had not received a copy of the result so was uninformed) to let her know the outcome. Back came the reply almost at once to bring forward my appointment to see her as soon as we were back from the Isle of Wight.

I spent the whole week's holiday worried sick but trying not to show it so as not to worry Phil. I expect he was just as worried but did not want to alarm me, so we dutifully did not talk about it much and carried on as though everything was all right. At my appointment at the Cambridge Nuffield on October 2nd, the oncologist ordered another blood test and a CT scan of the neck and chest to check for secondaries. The blood test at the Nuffield would be sent to Cardiff to be assessed, which was a different destination to where the blood test at the Pathology laboratory at work had been sent to. I was scanned, had blood taken, and went home to worry.

Having heard nothing after a couple of weeks, I emailed the Oncologist to ask if any secondaries had been found on the CT scan. Almost immediately she phoned me to say that she and the radiologist had been poring over my scans all afternoon, and unfortunately they could see small secondary spots on the lungs. Yes it was 'disappointing' that this had happened, and I would need another dose of radioactive iodine to hopefully put it right. This time I would have to come off my thyroxine tablets beforehand to ensure the treatment would be effective. This put the idea in my mind that perhaps the second treatment with the thyrogen had not been as effective as becoming hypo, and had caused the cancer to spread. She told me that many patients with secondary thyroid cancer were still alive 30+ years later, as being slightly over-medicated on thyroxine suppressed the thyroid stimulating hormone and stopped the lung secondaries from growing. She would book me into the Radioiodine Suite at Addenbrooke's for another ablative dose in the near future.

She also mentioned the latest thyroglobulin result was 0.5. I could not understand the discrepancy, and made a mental note to ask her why on my next appointment on December 4th. I put the phone down and broke the news to Phil, and we both sat looking at each other with tears in our eyes. We knew it was serious this time – the cancer had spread to the lungs. I told him if and when I was terminal and my body could not take any more, that I wanted to go to the Dignitas clinic in Switzerland where they practiced euthanasia as I did not want to suffer. He looked as devastated as I felt.

Meanwhile I had to go back to work and tell everybody that I now had secondaries and would need a month off work for more treatment. I would need to switch back to T3's for a month, and then stop taking any thyroxine tablets at all for two weeks prior to the start of my treatment on December 11th. I would become 'hypo' again. I remembered the aching legs, the puffy face and tired eyes and felt very depressed for the first time in a long time. Everyone at work was very kind, but I hated being different. I wanted to be normal and to do what everybody else did; to get up, go to work, come home and cook dinner etc; not the constant round of hospital visits and doctors' surgeries. News quickly spread around the workplace (a hospital grapevine is very efficient) and I was suddenly the talk of the office. I told my manager that my last day at work would be Friday 24th November, because on the following Monday I would be taking no thyroxine tablets and would feel too tired to work. I would not be back at work until Tuesday January 2nd 2007.

I also decided to ask the original endocrinologist who saw me in December 2004 for my notes and ultrasound scan reports. I wanted them to refer to as I was in the process of writing this book. I rang him at home after a few emails had produced nothing. He was worried there was going to be a complaint, but could hardly refuse me the notes as they were mine anyway. Eventually a couple of weeks later the notes arrived but not the ultrasound reports, as he informed me that the radiologist would have to give his permission for me to have them. After consulting with colleagues and confirming that I was entitled to have them, they were eventually faxed to me from the Bury Nuffield after some interjection by a senior work colleague.

October 2006 saw me moping around the house and trying to be cheerful at work, but feeling desperately sad. I felt my life was to be cut short and I was not ready to die. I wanted to see my granddaughter grow up, to see how the boys' jobs progressed, and I wanted to see how Matt's band fared. They had already won a band competition locally after only two months of playing together, and they showed so much promise. I realised I had inherited the cancer gene from one or both parents, and wondered if I was going to die at the same early age as my father. By the time he was my age, he only had a few months left of life.

One morning at work I was pushing my trolley of medical notes down to Medical Records. My chin was down and I felt that trying to carry on a normal life was meaningless when I was going to die anyway. What was the point? I had been to the medical library and looked up secondary thyroid cancer. Survival rates were as low as 50%. With cumulative doses of radioactive iodine, there was a chance of getting leukaemia as well if you had had more than 18,500 Becquerels (I had had about 9000 so far). But as I pushed the trolley down the corridor, I was suddenly overcome with a strange but very strong feeling that somehow everything was going to be okay. I suddenly felt lighter in mood but did not know why. It was only sometime later that I realised the feeling I experienced was when I was walking past the chapel. I am not in any way religious and cannot give any explanation for it, but in the depths of my misery I wondered if by a miracle I was going to survive.

Back at home I called out for some sort of sign that I would be okay (I do believe in the spirit world and have received messages from many mediums proving there is a spirit world). My call was answered within a very short time by a lightbulb popping out of its socket in the electric fire, which it had never done before. The bulb was still working when Phil put it back in. When lying awake in bed one night, I opened my eyes to put the light on to get a drink, and there was somebody sitting on the edge of my bed smiling. She had a white coat on and she looked like my oncologist. She stayed there for a couple of seconds before disappearing.

I clutched at straws. These were signs. I was going to be okay. I decided to book my meniscectomy operation for the period prior to coming off the thyroxine tablets so that I would only need to take one lot of sick leave and hopefully all my problems would be sorted at the same time. I was suddenly infused with hope. I explained all to the oral surgeon who could see I was still fit and he said it would not be a problem to do the operation (the oncologist had also said it would be ok). He would book me in for Thursday 23rd November 2006 at the Nuffield hospital at Ipswich. I asked him to take the troublesome crowned tooth out as well, which had become a huge abscess. Bacteria had got in whilst the temporary crown was on, and no antibiotic would touch it. He agreed, and I said a temporary goodbye to my work colleagues on Wednesday 22nd November. I hoped I felt recovered enough from the meniscectomy before I stopped the thyroxine T3 tablets on Monday November 27th.

CHAPTER 19 – MENISCECTOMY OF LEFT JAW

Thursday November 23rd saw Phil and I waiting in room 6 at the Ipswich Nuffield for my operation. Unfortunately I was last on the list (as usual) because I was the 'tricky' one. When the nurse had come in to take my temperature, she informed me it was high. I tried to tell her it was sometimes on the high side due to being over-medicated on thyroxine, but I was sure she thought I had an infection.

The anaesthetist had been to see me and had been informed of my locking jaw, secondary lung cancer, and the tendency for my heart rate and blood pressure to rise considerably after procedures involving a general anaesthetic. I imagined him throwing up his hands in horror and running away. He looked at my previous anaesthetic chart from July, but could see no real problems as the blood pressure and heart rate always settle down once I am asleep. He seemed very calm and confident and his attitude helped me to remain relatively calm. Perhaps I was not too much of a freak after all. Matt telephoned during the morning, but I could not tell him much as I was still waiting.

Finally at noon I was informed Theatre was ready for me. I dutifully got into bed in my gown and anti-DVT stockings, and hoped for the best. In the anaesthetic room a cannula was put in my hand and a sedative injected into it. A blanket came down over my brain and I remember no more until waking up in Recovery about an hour and a half later. I could hear somebody saying that I was 'tachycardic' but I remember thinking that I usually am after operations anyway. There was a swab in my mouth catching any remaining blood from the tooth extraction (thank goodness I had finally seen the last of lower right seven) and what felt like a very tight turban on my head with something hanging off of it. I asked for a drink but was refused as it was too soon. I was told that now I was awake I could be taken back to my room.

Phil was waiting yet again for me to come back. I wanted to feel what was hanging off the turban, but he put my hand down and said it was just a drain held in place by bandages (so that was what the turban was). It hurt to try and open my mouth, so I thought it best not to try. The nurse asked if I was in any pain, but thinking about it, it only hurt when I opened my mouth, so I said I didn't need any painkillers as the pain was not constant. Everybody seemed amazed. I was hoping I did not become nauseous, as it would be excruciatingly painful to be sick. I had remembered to ask the anaesthetist for a good anti-sickness injection and it seemed to have done the trick.

Phil gave me sips of water. I slowly came round and was thankful it was all over. Phil helped me to the toilet (what more could you want from a husband!) and I slowly started moving about. Now I just needed to recover enough before the radioiodine treatment in a couple of weeks' time.

I was discharged the next day after the nurse had taken the drain and cannula out, and had taken the turban off (what a relief to be free from that). There was a long scar going from just in front of my ear and up into my hairline. My hair had been shaved above my ear, and that was the worst bit as far as I was concerned! I had lots of stitches that would need taking out on Tuesday December 5th (my next appointment with the oral surgeon). I had a red rash on my face and chest that appeared in the car going home, but I knew that was the effect of the anaesthetic so did not worry about that too much. After my thyroidectomy, my face had changed to a brown colour and little rashes had appeared and disappeared, so I knew it was my body objecting to the anaesthetic in the only way it knew how. I did not know if the operation had been a success as it would probably be a week or so before I could open my mouth (if the last jaw operation was anything to go by), but I had a feeling this time the operation would work. Before I left the hospital the surgeon informed me he had never seen a disc so shredded. I had excelled myself in the realms of meniscus maceration.

Matt turned 21 during my recovery period. There was a party arranged at Cambridge on Saturday 25th November, but I did not feel well enough to go. Phil attended and said it all went off very well. I would have to wait for Anna's parents' New Year's Eve party instead. It looked to be a good night. I would be in charge of the music, and there would be fireworks at midnight in the garden. Evening dress was essential. I could not wait. It would be a chance to wear the expensive evening dress I had bought for the Caribbean cruise the year before. I would have to get my hairdresser to try and cut my hair so the two sides above my ears looked equal. At the moment it was rather lopsided; I was bald on one side and normal on the other.

After a week of recovery, I knew the operation had worked. There was no loud clicking when I opened my mouth, and my jaw had stopped locking. It had all been worth it. Awesome! I did not even mind another six weeks of pureed food again, because this time I could see an end to it all. The kitchen staff went out of their way this time not to give me anything with milk powder in it, and I was fine.

Matt's 21st birthday party

(Matt 2nd from left with band members & girlfriends)

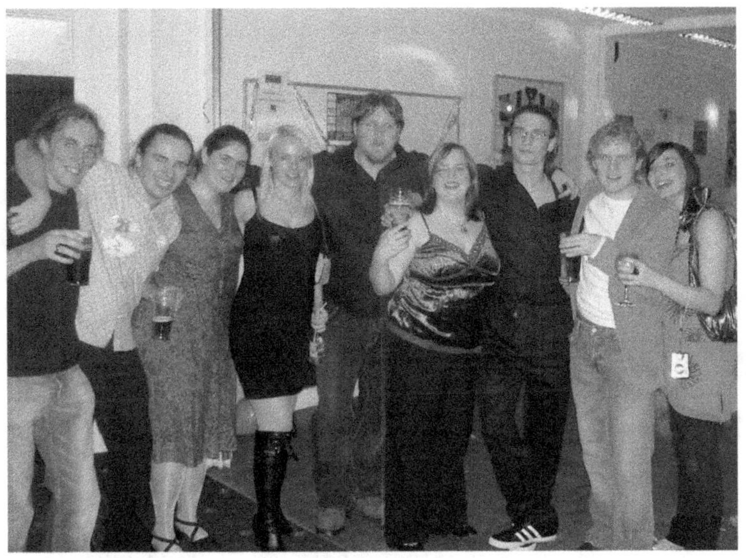

CHAPTER 20 – THIRD RADIOACTIVE IODINE TREATMENT

I had an appointment with the oncologist on Monday 4th December. By then I had been hypo for a week and was feeling cold (very unusual for me!) tired, and achy. I had also picked up what I thought was a slight chest infection from somewhere. The oncologist could not really tell me the outcome of the RAI treatment – whether it would kill the secondaries or not; I suppose she did not know herself. All she could tell me was that she knew some patients where it had worked (she presumably knew of patients where it had not worked, but was not saying).

Apparently, secondaries do not usually grow if they are suppressed with enough thyroxine. She had checked with eminent London oncologists as to my treatment, and had been reassured that everything was being done that could be done. Apparently I was making thyroglobulin antibodies which complicated matters somewhat (about 20% of thyroid cancer patients do this). My personal marker which would show either the cure or advancement of my cancer was to be the amount of thyroglobulin antibodies in my blood, and not the amount of thyroglobulin. The thyroglobulin result of 10.2 had been sent from the processing laboratories at Birmingham, and usually my oncologist would have sent it off to the laboratories at Cardiff. She said different laboratories either overestimated or underestimated the result. She said a result from Cardiff would have been lower. I would be having another blood test the following week in the RAI room before the start of the treatment, and presumably another one at a later date, and a scan at the end of the week as usual when the radiation levels in my body were at a safe dose. Hopefully the spots on my lungs would show up on the scanner, which meant they had taken up the RAI. We made another appointment for me to come back on 15th January 2007 for the results of the scan and blood tests.

I decided I was not going to worry about it all over Christmas – what will be will be. What I was looking forward to was the next day (Tuesday 5th December) when the stitches in my jaw were due to come out. I had an appointment with the oral surgeon at 2.25pm.

After my stitches had come out on the Tuesday, I started feeling quite ill with what I thought was a chest infection. Because I was hypothyroid, the phlegm was so thick and slow moving, that on a couple of occasions it lodged in my windpipe preventing me from breathing in properly. I had had to try and take a big breath in and cough it up. It was very scary, and I did not think I would be well enough to have the radioiodine dose. I phoned the oncologist on the Friday and she suggested I come into Addenbrooke's and have some tests to check for infection. My heart sank. Surely I had not taken all this time off work and got this far to be told it wasn't going to happen?

Phil and I arrived at the Radioiodine Suite on the Friday evening 8th December. The oncologist had arranged a chest x-ray and blood tests for me, and the nurses put me on antibiotics and a nebuliser at regular intervals. She also had the ENT surgeon who I had seen regarding my voice to look down my throat and see if all was well. He could not see anything too untoward, just lots of secretions going down the back of my nose. The blood results came back that it was not a chest infection, and therefore I would be well enough to undergo the treatment. Just being hypo had slowed down the phlegm production (as indeed it slows everything else down as well), but it was making me feel quite unwell in the process.

I stayed in for five nights eventually, and had my treatment on the Monday morning. During the Monday night I felt quite sick and panicked that I might vomit and injure my jaw. I quickly popped an anti-sickness pill and thankfully the feeling wore off. I wondered how much more my body could cope with. It really was turning out to be a massive endurance exercise. Also my eyes were not focusing due to being hypo – as if I needed any more things wrong with me.

By the Wednesday the radioactive iodine levels were low enough for me to go home. I hobbled out of Ward A5 and wondered how I was going to stay awake long enough to get to the car. I'd had no proper sleep since arriving at Addenbrooke's due to the phlegm problem, and also due to the bed being very uncomfortable. During the ride home I drifted in and out of sleep and worried about having to lie flat for the scan on the Friday, as it would be quite uncomfortable with the amount of phlegm at the back of my throat. The physicist had mentioned my worries to the scan technicians, and they apparently told him they would do their best to accommodate me. They could do the scan in sections so that I could be propped up. As it turned out, they did not even ask me if I wanted propping up; they just left me to get on with it and use mind over matter. It was a most uncomfortable 15 – 20 minutes.

My legs did not recover as quickly after re-starting the thyroxine as they had the first time. It took a good week for the achy calves to go, and for me to be able to stay awake for any length of time. I was determined to enjoy Christmas and not worry about if the treatment had worked or not. I hoped that after all I had suffered it would work, but secretly had some doubts.

CHAPTER 21 – AFTERMATH OF TREATMENT

Christmas Eve saw Phil, Mum, and I at Anna's parents' house for a get-together. The thyroxine levels were slowly coming up again and I was feeling a little better. The phlegm problem was still there, but at least it wasn't catching in my windpipe any more. Christmas Day lunch was in the Spread Eagle in Bury St Edmunds with Matt, Anna and Mum. Lee, Sarah and Sophie came to see us in the afternoon to exchange presents. There was some good news – I was going to be a grandmother again; baby number 2 was due 27th August 2007! Lee also joined us for lunch on 28th December at The Rushbrooke Arms in Sicklesmere when Mary, Dave, and Jenny came for a visit.

It was a great New Year's Eve party at Anna's parents' house. I danced until midnight and then felt really tired and wanted to go home. We had some gatecrashers who came in the front door, did a conga around the room, and then disappeared out the back door into the garden never to be seen again. Goodness knows where they went!

I was on tenterhooks when my appointment with the oncologist came around on January 15th. I told Phil I wanted to go on my own. I didn't want to put him through any more upset in case it was bad news.

No uptake was shown on the Gamma scan. The oncologist explained that it probably meant that the spots were too small to show up. I secretly thought it probably meant that the treatment had not worked, but decided to go along with her explanation as it offered more hope. She said she was going to give the radioactive iodine a few months to work, then I would need another blood test in May to check thyroglobulin antibody levels, and then another CT scan in early June to see if the spots were still there. Another appointment was made with her for July 2nd to obtain the results. It would mean another six months of waiting, but there was no other way round it. I came away disappointed and frustrated at the long wait to find out if I was going to be cured or not.

The phlegm problem persisted and would not go away (I had been told that there had been uptake of radiation in the back of my nose – hence the cause of the problem). My salivary glands became sore and painful during March and both problems carried on through spring and summer (the phlegm actually took at least 8 years before it went away!). The ENT surgeon prescribed a nasal spray and some pills to thin out the phlegm. It worked slightly and the phlegm became a little thinner, but unfortunately did not dry up completely. My mouth and throat were constantly dry due to the salivary glands not working properly, and I had to sip water all day, which eased the problem. I carried on at work but became tired of being asked the eternal question 'When will you be getting your results'? People were either trying to be kind and caring, or were just nosey – I could not decide which.

CHAPTER 22 – RESULT OF CT SCAN

It was a wonder the whole of the Nuffield Hospital could not hear my heart beating as I sat in the oncologist's office in July to hear my results. She said she could not see any lung secondaries on the scan, but sometimes it was difficult to see them if they were very small, and there were two small nodules in the lungs that had not changed from the previous scan. She also said that the scan showed two enlarged lymph nodes in my neck, which had got bigger since the first CT scan. She had not mentioned them the previous time, as she wanted to wait to see if the lung secondaries had enlarged. If they had not, then it would be worth giving me an operation (a left-sided neck dissection) to remove the lymph nodes. If the lung secondaries had become larger, then it would not have been worth putting me through the operation as I would have been terminal. So, at least I knew I was not terminal, but I would rather have been kept informed of my condition.

She told me the ENT surgeon who I had been seeing for my lack of voice and for the phlegm problem would do the neck dissection. I would receive an appointment to see him in the post. Swings and roundabouts – life gives with one hand and takes away with the other. I felt pleased that the lung spots had not enlarged, but disappointed that I would have to have yet another operation. I thought hard and decided it would be a good idea to have the operation at the end of

August. Then I would be recovered before Phil and I had our joint 50th birthday celebration party on October 13th, and then also I would be able to enjoy our holiday to St Lucia in November. There were also some music festivals mid –August which Matt's band were due to play in, and we had already booked tickets for these. Matt had also secured a better job with Marshall Aerospace in Cambridge which paid him another £9,000 per year. I was also due to become a granny again as Sarah's caesarean was due on 14th August. They had chosen the name Caitlin Marie for the new baby. I told the ENT surgeon that I would be ready for the operation on August 30th. By then there would be nothing left to look forward to except a Rush concert on October 6th. I sat in the car with Phil afterwards and cried.

The days passed slowly. Baby Caitlin being born helped to divert my thoughts for a while. The operation seemed to be on my mind the whole time. I wondered how the phlegm problem would affect me during the op; whether it would catch in my windpipe when I was unconscious. I resolved to mention the problem to the anaesthetist on the day. Food also seemed to get stuck sometimes, but a way round this problem I found was to eat slower and have smaller mouthfuls.

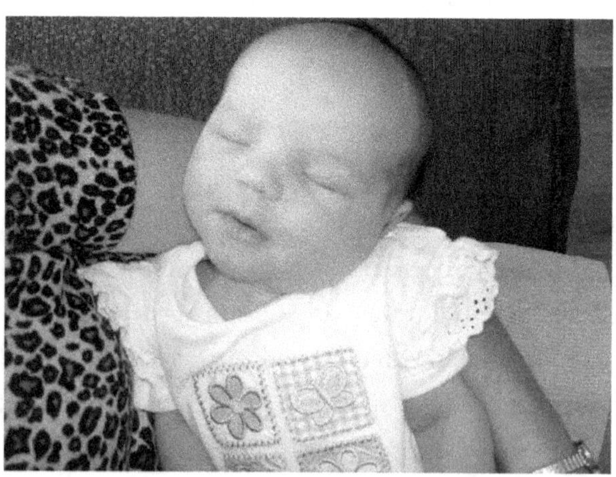

Baby Caitlin Marie born 14/8/07

CHAPTER 23 – NECK DISSECTION

Thursday 30th August came around far too quickly. Phil drove me to the Cambridge Nuffield, and we arrived about 12.30. The staff seemed very kind and helpful. I was given the usual gown and TED stockings to put on, and was told my operation would be at about 3pm. I was visited by the anaesthetist and I told him of the phlegm problem. He did not seem to think this mattered too much, and said he would 'look after me'. The surgeon came to see me beforehand too to take my consent and list all the things that could go wrong (pain, bleeding, infection, numbness, frozen shoulder, abnormal tongue movement, and difficulty in swallowing), and I mentioned the phlegm problem again.

I had also visited the Thyroid Cancer Support group online and had been reading the latest messages. One person who had had a neck dissection also had my voice box problem. When she vomited after the operation, the aspirant went down the windpipe and she had spent three days coughing it up. I had not vomited since before the original thyroidectomy, so had no idea if this would happen to me. The surgeon reassured me and said this was unlikely. If my throat had been open that much, then food and drink would go down the windpipe as well. I thought about it and was slightly reassured. There were also the usual visits from the doctor to put the cannula in, and one of the nursing staff to admit me and go through my medications.

Finally it was time to go. I actually walked with a nurse and Phil to the Theatre at 3pm. There I was met by the anaesthetist. I laid down on the trolley and said goodbye to Phil. I felt the anaesthetic go into the cannula and up my arm, then do not remember any more until waking up rather groggy in Recovery. I remember feeling extremely hot, and heard the nurse saying that I was tachycardic. It's the usual problem I get after operations – the heart rate and blood pressure go up for a couple of days. I was also aware that my heels hurt very much from lying flat for a length of time on the operating table.

As soon as I was awake, I was taken back to my room. Phil had been rather worried as I had been gone for about six hours. The surgeon came in to say that he had taken all the lymphatic tissue out on the left hand side of the neck (the right side at that time had been unaffected), and that after he had finished he could not see anything sinister left on that side in the neck. He said there had been a number of enlarged lymph glands, and also a very enlarged one down in the old thyroid bed which were now all gone. He said I might need some more radioactive iodine to kill any stray cells, and also the right side of the neck may or may not need attention in the future. I asked why the radiation the previous December had not killed all these glands, and the surgeon said that was because they were too big (the radiation works better on small pieces of tissue). I had two drains in, and would not be allowed home until these had been taken out. There was a big waterproof dressing covering the front of my neck and up to my left ear. I felt surprised to be still alive and that no phlegm had gone down the windpipe.

Over the next couple of days I tried to get out of bed. At first poor old Phil had to bring the bedpans in again, as they had inserted another cannula in Theatre for fluids and I was weeing for England again. Once again he did not shirk his duties, and hurried back and forth emptying them. On the second day I managed to get out of bed and use the commode which was an improvement on the bedpans. My back hurt, and on looking, Phil could see there was a graze which had not been there before the operation. Very mysterious! The nurse dressed it and reported it to Matron.

I was glad that I still had my coughing mechanism, which had been lacking after the thyroidectomy. The phlegm after that operation was much worse than this one, as I had not been able to cough it up. I had a couple of nebulisers as suggested by the nurse, but this time it did not seem too bad. The only thing I noticed on the second day was a tingling in my hands and face and tongue. I wondered if my parathyroid glands had been affected, but the doctor said wait and see if things settled down first. On the third day the tingling went, so that was a relief. The reversing agent that I had been given in Theatre to wake me up stayed in my system for quite a few days after. Every time I nodded off to sleep, then my brain woke me up straight away, as had happened with the thyroidectomy. It was awful.

On the Saturday one of the drains was taken out and the remaining one the day after. I was allowed to go home on the Sunday to recover. The nurse changed the dressing before I left, and said not to be too shocked at all the staples in my neck when I saw them. When Phil put a clean dressing on at home, he also told me not to look at the wound until all the staples were out. I decided to hold him to this, and therefore had no idea how it looked, but it must have looked bad.

Secretly I did look though, when Phil had gone back to work the next week and I was left at home to recover. I pulled the dressing back and yes it did look hideous, but I thought at the time how neat all the staples looked, stretching in a long line from my ear down to the middle of my neck. This surgeon knew his business, I thought. I was rather glad all the skin was numb surrounding the scar, because then it would not hurt too much when the staples were all taken out on the following Thursday. I seemed to be in continual pain in an area just below the scar on my chest. My neck and shoulder were stiff and sore and the skin was numb to the touch; indeed I couldn't move my head to the left at all. My left shoulder felt as though the surgeon had cut a big gouge along the top of it and then left it open and raw. When Phil took me to the GP surgery to have the staples removed, the nurse noticed the scar looked a bit red and called the doctor to have a look at it. The doctor agreed and put me on an antibiotic just to make sure it did not become too infected.

The pain was still there (although a little less) when I went to see the surgeon three weeks later for my check-up. He said there was nothing to worry about – I was bound to be in pain and it, plus the numbness, would go in time. He stressed I had to move my neck as much as I could otherwise it could become permanently stiff. He said results of the biopsy showed that 25 lymph glands had been removed and the majority of them had been cancerous, but at the end of the operation he had not seen any sinister-looking lymph nodes left. I would need another CT scan in three months' time to check there were not any enlarged glands left, and lifelong follow-up scans thereafter. He did not think the radioactive iodine worked on me particularly well, so it would have to be surgery in the future for any suspicious lumps that arose. He thought I would have a normal lifespan, but this type of cancer, although slow-growing, could come back at any time and therefore I might need more surgery. He checked my voice box with the camera just to make sure that my right vocal cord was still working: it was!

CHAPTER 24 – I MADE IT TO 50 AGAINST ALL ODDS!

Altogether I was off work for five weeks. It was a bigger operation than the original thyroidectomy, so took a little longer to recover from. The surgeon did say that it would take about six to nine months for the numbness to go, so I returned to work still feeling numb and a bit sore. I still had to cope with the phlegm problem as well, but it was not as bad as it had been earlier in the year. Also my eyes had been affected by the previous year's radiation and were watery and often infected. I had to carry Fucithalmic eye ointment around all the time.

Fortunately I was still able to enjoy the joint 50th birthday party that I had organised for Phil and myself on October 13th, one week after my return to work. I had a lovely time and danced for most of the night. I had made it to 50. I was very happy being surrounded with family and friends, and it made a lovely change from hospitals and doctors. My cousin Phillip had even come over from Saudi Arabia for the occasion, and made us a huge cake, which could have fed the entire village.

The week after that was another party to celebrate Anna's 21st birthday. This time Phil had to dress in his dinner suit, and I had had to scour the shops to find a 20's flapper dress, as the party had a 20's theme. Again I danced most of the night. I was partying for England even though I still could not move my neck very well. A couple of weeks after this Phil and I flew to St. Lucia for a well earned holiday. We stayed at the Sandals resort in Halcyon Bay in Castries. The sun shone, we lazed on the beach, and my scar healed slowly. It was bliss.

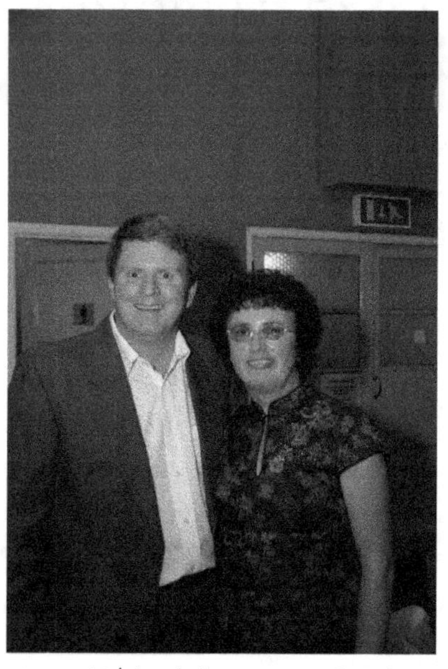

Phil and I at our joint 50th birthday party – October 2007. I searched through my wardrobe to try and find a high-collared top to cover the scar up on the night.

Back at home in December it was time for the three month scan. The skin surrounding the scar was still numb. The CT scan itself was not too bad – the only part I did not like was when the dye was injected. It made me feel very hot, but did not last for too long. Also part of the process of scanning the neck and chest involved holding my breath which was not too pleasant either, but I could cope with that.

Two weeks after the scan on December 17th I faced the ENT

surgeon who had performed the neck dissection. My heart was racing in dread of the possible results. He was smiling so I figured it could not be too bad. There were a couple of tiny nodes which he was going to keep an eye on, but all in all it was not too bad. The nodules in the lungs still had not changed, and he was not sure whether there was an enlarged lymph gland near my left ear, or whether it was muscle tissue. As far as I could tell, it was a case of looking at the next CT scan results in a year's time to see if anything changed and if so, where they went from there, and to take another blood sample to see if the thyroglobulin antibodies had reduced any. At least I did not need any more operations in the near future, and I still was not terminal. Oh well, at least I could enjoy Christmas!

This year we were all invited for Christmas dinner at Anna's parents' house in Ipswich. We provided the turkey and it was lovely sitting round a big table on Christmas Day with Matt, Anna, and all her family. They even invited my mother to share in the celebrations. Boxing Day saw everyone at our house for a get-together, and then it was back to Anna's parents on New Year's Eve for a party to see in 2008. Perhaps it would be next year when I would be finally rid of this dreadful disease.

CHAPTER 25 - 2008

The New Year started off with a visit in early January to London Theatreland to see Phantom of the Opera. I loved it so much that I vowed to go again before too long.

I also decided to make an appointment at the Eye Clinic at the hospital where I worked to find out why my eyes were always watery and why they often became infected. I was told I had blepharitis, an inflammation of the eyelids, and this was probably not caused by the radioactive iodine as I had first thought. I was told to wash the eyes thoroughly with hot water every morning and evening, which would help to clear any dirt and debris, the likely causes of this irritating condition. Strangely enough this did seem to help a little bit, but did not take away the problem altogether.

January 2008 was also the time when I decided to enrich my mind and began to learn Pitman 2000 shorthand. Eight months later I still had not progressed very far, but it did stretch my middle-aged mind trying to remember all the little lines, dots, and squiggles. I also signed on at work for an NVQ Level 3 in Business Admin. It was all free and so why not?

On February 18th it was time for another check-up with the ENT surgeon who had performed my neck dissection. I still had no feeling on the left side of my neck, and if I faced frontwards and moved my head over to the right, it felt very peculiar indeed. Still; the scar had healed well, and he could not detect any new lumps or bumps in my neck, which was all to the good. I still had phlegm problems at the back of my throat, and sometimes food became stuck if I did not eat carefully, but on the whole things were improving. He said the blood test performed in December did show a slight reduction in thyroglobulin, but it was not really worth me having further blood tests as the antibodies I made rendered tests mostly non-viable. They would concentrate mainly on the results of CT scans to plan further treatment. It seemed that radioactive Iodine was not very successful either, so as far as I could see only surgery would be available to me as a treatment should the cancer progress.

Another check-up was due three months hence, and another scan was due in December. I felt well enough, was enjoying work, and also was relieved no further surgery was needed at that time. Phil and I had a nice week off work in March and visited Old Trafford football ground for a tour (part of Phil's Christmas present from me), and had a boat ride up the Thames from Greenwich culminating in a ride on the London Eye.

I had decided just before Christmas it was time for me to again try to stop the norethisterone tablets that regulated my periods and had thankfully eradicated my PMT problems for the past 12 years. I was 50 now and surely I must be pre-menopausal? All my old school friends were going through the menopause, as I had found out when we attended their 50th birthday dinners in April and May. A few months off the tablets to get the norethisterone out of my system and then a blood test would show whether I should consider HRT or not. I did not feel menopausal though, and by February it was clear that coming off the tablets was giving me some 'interesting' side effects (but we won't go there!).

It was no good though – the terrible PMT symptoms had returned by May, and I could not wait to have the blood test done and start taking the tablets again. The blood test showed normal levels. I was not menopausal, so before you could say 'hot flushes' I was back on the norethisterone tablets. The GP assured me that I would know when I was menopausal, as norethisterone is progesterone only, so the tablets would not stop the dreaded hot flushes when they occurred, only oestrogen would do that. It was a terrible mistake coming off the norethisterone, as my body seemed to produce too much oestrogen and I did not seem to have the progesterone to counterbalance it. I must be the only middle aged woman in the world who is actually looking forward to the menopause. I try and get by without taking tablets if at all possible, but norethisterone and thyroxine are the two I cannot do without!

The blood test had also shown that my eosinophil count was raised. I quickly contacted my oncologist, who assured me that as I suffered from hayfever and it was the hayfever season, this was the reason that the eosinophil count had risen to 1.7. She asked me to have another blood test in August after the hayfever season had finished, to see if it had decreased any. I was reassured by this, as I had read on the Internet that it could be a sign of leukaemia. Perhaps I read too much.

May 2008 was also the time that Matt and Anna found a place of their own. They moved into rented accommodation in Cherry Hinton, and seemed extremely happy together. They had tired of sharing a house with five other students. Two of the students had very strange habits, would not talk to the others, and would share a bath at 2am. These two eventually married, but not before Matt and Anna had moved out. With a place of their own, Anna could at last have the parlour-grand piano that had belonged to her grandfather taken out of storage and deposited in their front room. Matt had one of the bedrooms as his music room, with all his amps and guitars set up to his liking. He was as happy as a pig wallowing in the brown stuff.

Another successful check up with the ENT surgeon occurred in May. There was nothing much to report. No lumps could be felt in my neck. He said the oncologist wanted to see me in August for a check-up, and then it would be back to him again in November for another check-up.

I also visited a world-renowned healer, Matthew Manning at his home near Bury St Edmunds** in May for the first of three healing sessions. He placed his hands on my neck for about 20 minutes to the accompaniment of soothing music. I had read that it had been scientifically proven that the force of his healing hands could change cancer cells in test tubes, and he had cured many people with cancer, including his own wife. If it worked I was all for it. I was doing all I could to help myself.

We were getting out and about with a couple of friends from work to see various bands. Matt's band were winding down after a very successful 2007, where they had played at a couple of big festivals. Two band members were leaving to go to University, and one band member left because he was fed up with it all. Phil and I bought tickets for the Isle of Wight Festival which was due to be held in June, and asked the lovely Betty if we could rent her bungalow again so that we didn't have to suffer the horrors of camping and using festival toilets in the middle of the night. We love going to the music festivals, and if we could not see Matt play, then we would set our souls free in the sunshine and join the beautiful people at Seaclose Park. We had to interrupt this idyll as we had been invited to attend Anna's brother Alex's wedding on the Saturday in Sudbury, but it was back on the ferry Saturday night to see The Police close the festival on the Sunday evening. Below is a photo of myself at the Isle of Wight festival in June 2008.

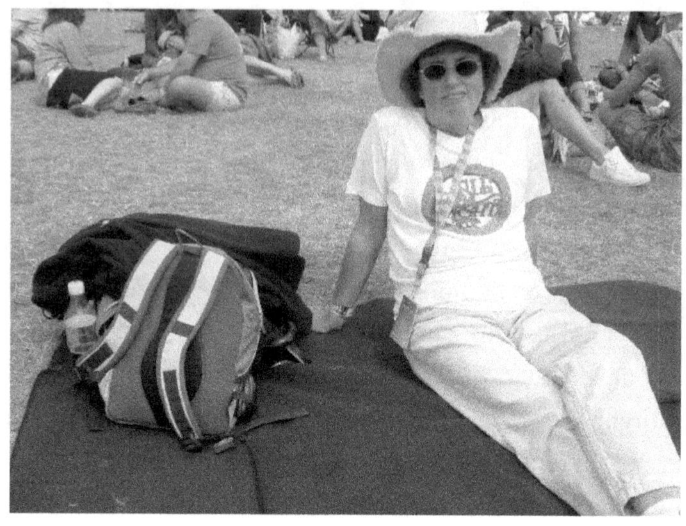

An unexpected bonus occurred in July. Phil booked a surprise weekend trip to Dublin for us. We flew from Stansted airport and stayed in the Temple Bar area. I dragged him around St. Fintan's graveyard looking for Thin Lizzy frontman Phil Lynott's grave (we found it after a long search), visited Oscar Wilde's house in Merrion Square, and enjoyed a Riverdance performance at the Gaiety Theatre. What a lovely weekend. There were walks along the banks of the Liffey, and also shopping in the famous Grafton Street. All too soon it came to an end, and it was back to work again on the Monday.

Two family birthdays occurred in July. Granddaughter Sophie was three, and our eldest son Lee was 26. Lee was now a service manager; no longer the air-conditioning apprentice doomed forever to make the tea and get the bacon torpedoes in. He has made a name for himself in the air-conditioning industry as one of the best engineers around. Matt at the tender age of 22 has recently been promoted to supervisor in his field as a CNC machine programmer. I was very proud of my ever-growing family, and wanted to be around for quite a few more years to see my granddaughters grow up.

**As an update, Matthew Manning now works at 'The Haven Health Clinic, 24 West Street, Ashburton, Devon, TQ13 7DU

CHAPTER 26 – ONE YEAR AFTER THE NECK DISSECTION

We had been invited to another wedding in August 2008. Mary and Dave's eldest daughter Clare was marrying her long-term partner Steve. She looked stunning in her dress on the day, and it was lovely to have all the family together and happy. I do like weddings. Unfortunately Lee and Sarah could not make the wedding, but Matt and Anna turned up for the evening reception and we danced the night away.

My youngest granddaughter Caitlin was one on August 14th, and Sarah organised a little party for her. The Monday following the party I was back at the Nuffield in Cambridge to see the oncologist for a check-up.

The oncologist was all smiles after she had felt around my neck, and assured me that my neck felt 'perfectly normal'. Thank goodness for that! She booked me in for a scan in December, and I had some blood taken to check for thyroglobulin levels, TSH, T3, and T4. She made an appointment for me to see her again on December 8th to get the results of the latest CT scan. All seemed well. The last blood test done a couple of weeks before at the GP surgery showed my eosinophil count had gone down to 1.3, so at the moment all was groovy in my little world.

About a month after the blood test, the results came in. My

thyroglobulin levels had reduced to 0.5, thyroglobulin antibodies had reduced to just under 500 (they had been near to 1000 the previous year), and TSH was less than 0.03. The neck dissection had been worth it. These results were all encouraging. The only downside was that my T4 level was 32 – too high! I would have to reduce my thyroxine dosage slightly. The oncologist suggested taking 125mcg of thyroxine on Mondays, Wednesdays, and Fridays, and 150mcg the rest of the week. There would be another blood test nearer Christmas when my scan was due to check if this new dose was right for me. I hoped I would not start putting on weight with the reduced dose, as up till now I had been able to eat what I wanted and still stay the same weight. However, if I had to have an operation where I had to be nil by mouth for a day, then I could lose half a stone in a day. Perhaps the thyroxine dose was slightly too high for me!

Whilst I had been waiting for the blood test results, something very unexpected happened. Matthew and Anna announced their engagement on September 3rd. They had been together for 6 years, so I suppose it was about time! I envisioned Anna's Mum and I having fun organising a big engagement party for them, and there would be another family wedding to look forward to in 2010. The setting had been quite romantic for the proposal. Matt had popped the question whilst they were on holiday with Anna's family in Canada. They were staying at her auntie's cottage on Bruce Beach, and he had waited until it was sunset and then had got down on one knee on the beach with a lovely engagement ring in his hand. Ah! Needless to say Anna said 'yes'! I now had two sons, two daughters – in-law, two granddaughters, one very lovely husband, and good blood results. What more could I want? My cup was running over as they say. To cap it all I had received a 'normal' result from my first routine mammogram which all women over 50 are encouraged to have, and another above average score for my age on a further bone density scan. It was nice to be 'normal' for a change.

There was also a break in Beaulieu Sur Dordogne, France, at the end of September. We had been invited to stay with the managing director of the company where Phil works and his wife in their house for a long weekend. After knowing them for over 20 years they were more like friends than employer and employee. They paid for our airfare, met us at the airport, and showed us the sights around their local area. Their house was more like a mansion, and boasted a large swimming pool, a cinema room, a bar and wine cellar, a pool/snooker room, and in fact anything you could possibly want. The weather was gorgeous for the end of summer, and we swam in the pool every day and ate from the barbeque on the large patio at night. We visited the huge market at Salat, the village and chapel carved from the rocks at Rocamadour, and a restaurant with stunning views over the valley and Dordogne River at Domme. At the end of our visit they took us back to the airport, making sure we had some lunch with us! What more could you want from your employers?

October 2008 saw me back at the GP surgery for a NHS re-referral to the Eye Clinic at the hospital where I work. No matter how I tried to stick to the instructions given to me the last time I attended when it was thought I had blepharitis, it made no difference. My eyes still became infected, sore and watery on now increasingly regular occasions, and I was becoming very tired of constantly having to wipe my watery eyes all the time. My eyes were also over-sensitive to light, causing me to always have to wear dark glasses when outside, and I always tried to avoid driving at night due to other cars' headlights being too dazzling. The GP informed me that patients with thyroid problems always seem to have eye problems as well, but he agreed with the ophthalmologist's last letter when he remarked that he thought my problems had nothing whatsoever to do with having three doses of radiation. He prescribed chloramphenicol ointment, which unfortunately did not work. I wondered how was it then that my eye problems only started after having the RAI treatment? An appointment was sent to me to attend the Eye Clinic on November 17th.

I mentioned the eye problem to my mother a few weeks before I was due to attend the clinic. She came up with the old-fashioned remedy of cleaning the eyes with a solution of sodium bicarbonate twice a day (a quarter of a teaspoon in cooled, boiled water). I tried that and it worked to start with, but found I still had eye infections from time to time, and my eyes still watered when I walked outside in a cold wind. Nothing really seemed to work. Another visit to a different GP ensued before the Eye Clinic appointment. This GP suggested using some baby shampoo in warm water and cotton buds to scrub the eyelids every day, as she was sure it was blepharitis. She also took a swab, as I had an eye infection at the time. I trawled the Internet in desperation and found a correlation between cumulative doses of RAI and a blockage of the eyes' drainage systems causing watery eyes and frequent conjunctivitis. Result! The condition is called epiphora, and I had all the symptoms. If it was found that I had this problem, then it could be cured with minor surgery. I would mention it at the Eye Clinic appointment.

The last of my three healing appointments occurred at the end of October. Matthew Manning informed me that I was 'as fit as a fiddle' and there was 'nothing wrong with me'. I had just bought two of his books and was reading about his childhood experiences with psychic phenomena. Like me, he had also experienced his bed moving as a young child, and I felt an affinity with him as I turned the pages (people do tend to look at you strangely when you mention something like this!). He did not ask me to make another appointment, but I said I might be in touch after my scan results in December (I like to keep my options open) if I was not given the all clear.

There was another successful check-up with the ENT surgeon on 10th November. He placed the well-hated scope in the right nostril again to check on the vocal cords and the back of the throat (my heart sinks when I see that scope). I had mentioned to him that very occasionally (about five times a year) food or phlegm would get stuck at the back of my throat making it difficult for me to breathe in, and I would have to cough very hard to dislodge it. To me it seemed as though my windpipe was blocked when this happened. He reassured me that the paralysed vocal cord was in quite a good position, and the back of my throat looked normal. Because of its position, there was not much that could be done to move the vocal cord to a position where the strength of my voice could be improved and to stop the windpipe being occasionally blocked. There was a risk that any operation performed could also make me permanently short of breath, with no real relief of symptoms. I told him I'd leave it. I realised this was the 'new normal' and I would have to live with it. He could feel no new lumps in my neck though, and said he did not need to see me again for six months. He said he would meet up with the oncologist to have a look at the CT scan which I was to have on 5th December. If any more enlarged lymph nodes showed up, he informed me that he could operate and remove them.

By now the effects of the reduced dose of thyroxine were beginning to kick in. I found I did not feel as hot as before, but unfortunately I had put on half a stone in weight. The temptation was to buy bigger trousers, but if I did that I would just be buying bigger and bigger ones as time went by, so I decided to cut down a bit on the Mr Kipling lemon slices, which fortunately never seemed to block my windpipe however many of them I ate.

At the end of November there was a lovely party at Abington Hall, Cambridge, to celebrate Matt and Anna's engagement. We danced all night, and met up with Mary and Dave, and Phil's nieces

Clare, with new husband Steve, and Jenny with her boyfriend, and nephew Paul. Matt and Anna had organised everything themselves including the music and a slideshow of old photos of them as babies. Lee and Sarah came along (having secured a babysitter at the last minute), and it was lovely to have all the family together.

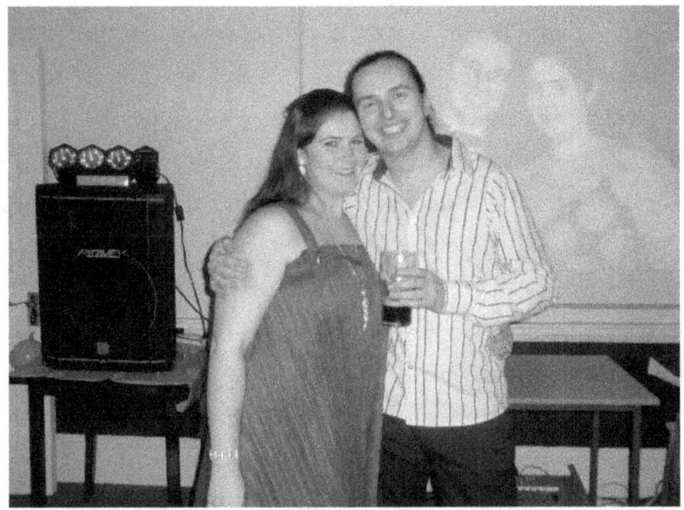

Matt and Anna at their engagement party – November 29th 2008.

The dreaded appointment with the oncologist came on the 8th December 2008 to get the results of a CT scan I had had three days previously. Walking into her office that morning after having no sleep for three nights due to worrying about what might be found, I was not feeling at my best. I had taken heart though from all the good wishes on Facebook from my family and friends, and was trying to think positively. The oncologist was quick to point out that nothing had changed since the last scan; the tiny lung spots were still there but had not grown due to their growth being suppressed with thyroxine, and the two slightly enlarged lymph glands in my neck that the ENT surgeon had mentioned after my previous scan a year before had not enlarged either, and were unchanged. The oncologist did also say that the two lymph glands might just be slightly enlarged anyway in their normal state, and possibly were not cancerous at all. As far as she could tell, I was in remission. All I needed was a blood test to check that my new thyroxine level was correct. I had mentioned the slight weight gain, but Phil and I picked up on the overall vibes that if the levels were correct I would just have to eat less (the gates of heaven are narrow I hear, and if I eat too many lemon slices I will not be able to get in when the time comes).

Such a relief! I was in remission! I had been waiting a long time to hear this. I had been given a new lease of life, and I was going to make the most of it. Phil and I walked back to the car that morning on cloud nine.

Also after mentioning my frequent eye infections and watery eyes to the oncologist, she sent an urgent faxed referral to a consultant ophthalmologist at the Nuffield hospital in Bury, and I would receive an appointment to see him two days later. I cancelled the NHS Eye Clinic appointment, as I knew it would be better to see a consultant, and I would not necessarily have seen one at my NHS appointment.

When the blood test result came back, it showed that the thyroid stimulating hormone level was raised too much. If I carried on with the reduced thyroxine dose, then probably the lung spots would start to grow. The oncologist quickly sent me instructions to go back to the original dose of 150mcg. There was an upside to this news though - I could now put Mr Kipling's lemon slices back on my weekly shopping list. Some more good news; the thyroglobulin level eventually came back as less than 0.5, and the thyroglobulin antibodies had reduced even more from September and were now 441.4.

Back at the Nuffield again for my eye appointment, the ophthalmologist measured the pressure in each eye (which was normal), and applied some yellow dye to check if the tear ducts were working – they were. He diagnosed recurrent follicular conjunctivitis, which he said was a non-bacterial infection probably caused by the radiation. It was the frequent infections that were making the tear ducts swollen and therefore narrower. He prescribed some steroid eye drops for me to take for two months to see if they stopped the infections. He told me not to use baby shampoo to clean the eyes with, but to stick to the sodium bicarbonate solution. I was to see him again for review after the two months were up. If the steroid did not work, then he would try something else. At last it looked as if the eye problems would soon be sorted out as well. What a wonderful Christmas it was going to be this year!

CHAPTER 27 – UPDATE
AT THE END OF 2008

So, after two major operations, three doses of radiation, and four years on from finding the original lump, how am I at the end of 2008? Because I have only one vocal cord I have a weak voice that is fine for day to day living, but put me in a room with loud music or loud background noise and I will struggle to make myself heard. I cannot read long passages aloud to my grandchildren without gasping for breath, and I cannot sing a song all the way through, as I cannot seem to breathe in fast enough to keep up, and also cannot reach any high notes. I am 'lucky' in that I did not have this affliction when my boys were small, as some degree of shouting had to be undertaken on my part on quite a frequent basis (the ENT surgeon does tell me though, that compared to his other patients with the same condition, my voice is one of the better ones).

Also, again probably because of the paralysed cord, food very occasionally becomes stuck in the back of my throat, making it rather alarming for fellow diners if I am out in a restaurant when this occurs. If I have a cold or cough, my voice is the first thing I lose and it is the last thing to return once the germ goes away. There is still a slight phlegm problem caused by the uptake of RAI at the back of my throat, which occurred during my last stay in Addenbrooke's RAI suite in November 2006, but it is slowly improving. My left jaw joint is not very robust and I have to avoid biting down on hard foodstuffs, but it does not lock any more. On a happier note, my eyes have not been as watery or infected since starting the steroid drops, so hopefully this problem will soon ease. The left side of my neck and top of my left shoulder remain numb, and probably always will be, and oh yes, I don't do heat.

Due to all that extra thyroxine pumping round, my body temperature is higher than everyone else's and I am hot quite a lot of the time. After living with me for nearly 30 years, Phil does not do heat either, and our visitors usually know to put extra jumpers on when they visit. Our faces are always redder than anyone else's, we have not got central heating, and could not think of anything worse than having to sit in a hot, stuffy room. We actually have an air-conditioning unit in our lounge instead (thanks Lee!), and cooling fans in every room that get used a lot in the summer months.

But hey, there are millions of people worse off than me. Working as a medical secretary and typing clinic letters for other people tells me that, and I am grateful to still be here to see my granddaughters growing up. I am looking forward to our cruise aboard the Royal Caribbean's ship 'Radiance of the Seas' in February 2009 which will visit various ports in South America and also stop for us to attend the Rio de Janeiro carnival, and I still aim to be around on 6th August 2010 for Matt and Anna's wedding day. Anna asked me to write a poem to be read on their special day, and I have included it below (only because they have already read it and approve!). I will ask Anna's brother, Alex, to read it out on the day, as the problems I have would make it impossible for me to project my voice across a large room.

TO MATT AND ANNA ON THEIR WEDDING DAY

1   Two brown soulful eyes,
A wise little face,
A new brother for Lee,
I look at Matthew
And he looks at me.

2   He's quiet and shy,
Where I go
There he'll be,
I cuddle Matthew
And he cuddles me.

3   Not keen on playgroup,
Doesn't want to learn,
Two sad brown eyes
Await my return.

4   First day at school
He's grown so tall,
He's made me a picture
To hang on the wall.

5   Now he goes to Upper school,
Runs for the bus so as not to be late,
Waves goodbye at the garden gate.
He visits friends who live near and far,
One day he sees my old guitar.

6   "Teach me some chords Mum",
The guitar's in his hand,
Before you know it,
He's joined a band.

7   He grows his hair
His friends aren't posh,
Some of them
Don't appear to ever wash.

8   "We need a Singer"
Who will it be?
I place some adverts.
We wait and see.

9   A girl replies,
She sends a text.
They arrange to meet
On Saturday next.

10   She arrives in a car
With her Father and Mother,
They've both come to see
Who's got his eye on their daughter.

11   Her Father jumps out
       Shakes Matt by the hand,
       Her Mother's less keen,
       Anna's only fifteen.

12   Matt has long hair, big boots,
       A leather jacket and all,
       Alison's phone is by her ear
       In case Anna has to call.

13   They walk and talk,
       The time flies by,
       Now Anna meets us
       Who are waiting nearby.

14   They walk towards us
       Hand in hand,
       That's quick work thinks I,
       It pays to be in a band.

15   She's a very sweet girl
       With long dark hair,
       She answered the advert
       For a dare.

16   My son is in love
       The world around him grows dim.
       He cuddles Anna,
       And she cuddles him.

17   And so it must pass,
       It's part of nature's plan,
       From mother to wife,
       Now he's grown to a man.

18   As we sit here today,
       I'll say to each and every one,
       I've gained a daughter,
       Not lost a son.

BOOK 2

2007 ONWARDS

CHAPTER 28 – 2009 AND
EYES NOT RIGHT

The symptoms had started in September 2007 soon after my neck dissection. Perhaps I was a bit run down after the operation, but a short time after I returned home from hospital I came down with conjunctivitis. I thought nothing of it, visited the GP surgery where a nurse prescribed Fucithalmic ointment, and the symptoms soon cleared up.

It was during the winter of 2007 when I noticed my eyes were watering every time I went outside in the cold wind. This new problem did not resolve with time, in fact it became worse. It eventually caused me to visit the eye clinic at the hospital where I work in early 2008 for an opinion. According to the ophthalmologist there I had blepharits, an inflammation of the eyelids, and all I needed to do was clean the eyes twice a day with a weak solution of Sodium Bicarbonate.

For a while this did work, but all too soon the watery eyes returned, along with more frequent infections. It was like looking through a net curtain when I had an attack; the eyes would be sore, oozing pus and itchy, and my vision would be cloudy. The condition was rather miserable to live with, and I'm sure my husband Phil was suffering right along with miserable me.

By the end of 2008 I was getting infections every couple of weeks, and my eyes were watering continually. The GP was about as much use as a chocolate fireguard; apparently thyroid disease and eye problems went hand in hand. I had Fucithalmic ointment on repeat prescription, and carried a sackful of tissues everywhere I went. This had to stop. I made a new patient appointment in December 2008 at the Bury St Edmunds Nuffield hospital to see another ophthalmologist after clearing it with my long-suffering insurance company.

This new ophthalmologist examined my eyes, said there was quite a bit of inflammation present, and prescribed FML (Fluorometholone) eye drops; a weak steroid. I was told to start off with four drops a day in each eye for two weeks, then three drops a day for a week, and finally two drops a day until he saw me again on February 12th 2009. We were due to go on a South American cruise on February 14th, sailing on the Royal Caribbean's cruise ship 'Radiance of the Seas'. One of the stops would be in Rio de Janeiro, where we were due to visit Corcovado Hill to see the statue of Christ the Redeemer, and also visit Sugar Loaf Mountain and of course attend the carnival of samba schools in the Sambadrome. I hoped the eye problem would be sorted by then.

What a delight! As soon as I started with the four drops of FML a day for the first fortnight all my symptoms disappeared, my eyes dried up, and all was well in my little world. Three drops per day for the third week had the same effect, and even dropping to two drops a day did not produce any of the previous symptoms. We'd cracked it at last!

The FML ointment ran out in early February, and unfortunately the infections and watering returned with a vengeance. Thank goodness I had a follow up appointment on February 12th.

I poured out my tale of frustration and woe to the ophthalmologist. He said I probably had not been taking the FML for long enough, and prescribed me some more to take for another two months. He said I did not need to come back any more, as taking two drops a day of the FML for a bit longer would banish the symptoms altogether. Result!

Off we headed to Heathrow on February 14th, with my precious eye drops tucked away safely in my handbag. We had a 2-hour flight to Madrid, a further 11 hour flight to Buenos Aires, and then an overnight stay in the City Tower hotel in Buenos Aires before we could board the ship on the Sunday morning. During the 11 hour flight it was time to apply some eye drops, so I thought I'd visit the loo and apply them in there. What I had not thought of was the effect the cabin pressure would have on my little container. As soon as I undid the cap and turned it upside down ready for application, the liquid almost squirted out instead of dripping out in tidy little drops. Oh dear, I lost quite a bit of it in the process. I hurriedly replaced the lid and decided to wait until I was at the hotel to have another go.

My eyes were fine for the first week of the holiday. The ship was a wonderful five-star floating hotel. The crew could not do enough for us – even folding our bath towels into animal shapes every day! It docked in several ports in Brazil before arriving at Rio at the start of the second week. Everyone was in carnival mood. Rio's streets are teeming with carnivals at that time of the year, but we were taken to the mother of all carnivals at the Sambadrome. Here is where the best 12 samba schools parade down the main route. Each school wants to win the main prize of half the gate money (the Sambadrome holds about 50,000 people) and the kudos that goes with it. The schools parade one at a time in front of judges, and they are allowed one hour to parade from one end of the main route to the other. Most of the schools consist of about 4000 people. If their carnival parade takes longer than one hour they lose points. Each parade begins with a firework display. The carnival parades take place over two nights, finishing around 6am the following day.

The heat inside the Sambadrome was stifling, even though it was 9pm at night when we arrived. The coaches were due to start taking us back to the ship at around midnight, so we would see at least two samba schools perform. We were shoulder to shoulder on the concrete steps. I accidentally touched Phil's leg and it was dripping wet. Ugh. I could not even move away as I had an equally sweaty person on the other side of me. I was doing a good job of perspiring myself, but had the foresight to bring along a little battery-operated fan. I think I would have melted into a puddle otherwise.

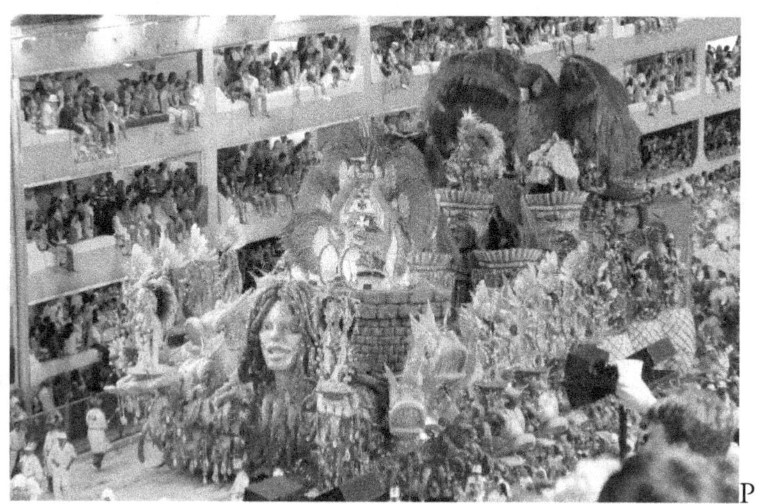

Photos shot from inside the Sambadrome.

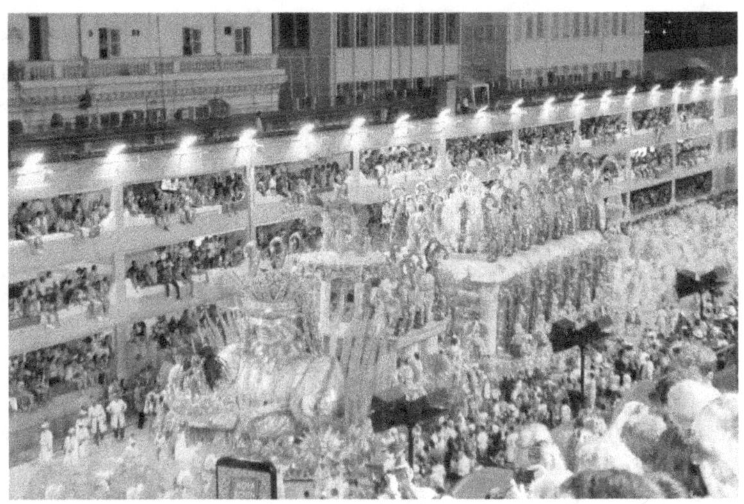

The carnival parades were fantastic though; it put our little annual carnival in Bury St. Edmunds to shame. The samba schools were all made up of poor local people who worked on their costumes all year round, and for them it was an honour to take part.

Whilst in Rio we also took the funicular railway up Corcovado Hill to see the statue of Christ the Redeemer in all its glory, and rode the cable car up Sugar Loaf Mountain. We did try to sit on Copacabana beach, but it was too hot. Everybody seemed to have brought his or her own parasol, and of course we did not have one and there did not seem to be any for hire. Bronzed lovelies in thongs walked nonchalantly by in the searing heat, and there we were sweating and frying in our T-shirts and shorts trying to find some shade!

After the ship left Rio, my eyes started watering again slightly. Thank goodness I did not have any infections on holiday, but the watery eyes had definitely started again. The drops had not even run out by the end of March, but the constant watering and infections had returned. I threw the drops away and decided to not only go back and see the ophthalmologist, but to also obtain a second opinion (once bitten twice shy). The ophthalmologist suggested that the strength of the steroid had probably not been strong enough. He prescribed very strong steroid drops namely Predsol Forte (Prednisolone), and a strong antibiotic, Ofloxacin. I was to take one drop of each in both eyes three times a day for three weeks. In his words it was time to 'attack the eyes with a shotgun instead of a pea-shooter'. He also said there was no surgical treatment for the condition.

Within hours of starting the new medication regime my symptoms cleared up entirely. What bliss! I was still infection-free the following week when I saw a new ophthalmologist (recommended by my oncologist) at the Cambridge Lea hospital for a second opinion.

CHAPTER 29 – A SECOND OPINION

The new ophthalmologist was very thorough. Again like the first specialist he examined my eyes, noted the pressure was slightly raised due to the steroid (it would take about six weeks to reduce back to normal after discontinuing it), but said he could see no infection or inflammation present (the steroid was doing its job). He said I would need to come back and see him when I did have an infection, as there was not much he could do with eyes that seemed perfectly normal. He agreed with the prescription for the strong steroid and antibiotic, but differed from the first specialist in that he thought there was a surgically remediable treatment if the steroid did not work; firstly to syringe the tear ducts, and then if that did not work to perform dacryocystorhinostomies. This is a procedure to bypass the blocked naso-lacrimal ducts under anaesthetic whereby a new opening for the ducts are made by chipping out a piece of bone at the top of the nose and creating a new drainage passage. I hoped I did not need it though.

He also said he would research my claim that the radiation had caused the tear ducts to narrow or block, thus stopping the tears from draining away properly and causing the watering and infection. He had never heard of radiation causing this problem, but was interested enough in my case to look into it. He actually did find a link between radioiodine (which gets concentrated in the tears) and narrowing of the tear ducts, which he was kind enough to detail in his clinic letter to me. It was wonderful to be believed.

I carried on with the short course of steroid and antibiotic and the eye problem stayed at bay. I was due to finish the course a day or so before we had a long weekend in the Lake District in early May, but I decided to carry on taking it just to make my weekend away the best it could be. I am a fan of Wordsworth's poetry, and we visited his childhood home at Cockermouth, and Dove Cottage and Rydal Mount near Grasmere, a couple of the homes he lived in with his family as an adult. There was also a visit to St. Oswald's Church at Grasmere where the Wordsworth family are buried, and trips by cruiser and a self-drive motor boat on Lake Windermere. I had never visited the Lakes before and could see why Wordsworth wrote such beautiful poetry whilst sitting in his summer house at Rydal Mount overlooking peaceful hills, valleys and lakes.

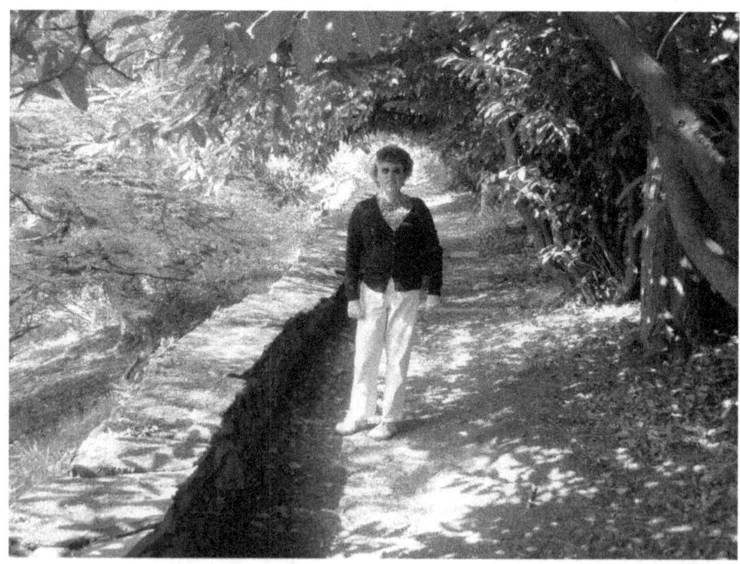

Myself in Wordsworth's garden at Rydal Mount.

A week or so after the visit to the Lakes it was time for my six-monthly check up with the ENT surgeon who had performed my neck dissection in August 2007. I alternated the check –ups with an oncologist I had been seeing since the diagnosis of papillary thyroid cancer in June 2005, so was not due to see her until the end of the year. I think they worked on the idea that two heads were better than one when it came to my check –ups and treatment options. The ENT surgeon felt my neck for any lumps (none found fortunately) and looked at my vocal cords using the camera-via-the-nostril approach (yet another unpleasant experience), and could see the left cord was still paralysed. He was sure he could help my voice become stronger by performing an operation whereby the vocal cords were pushed closer together, but at that moment I was happy with what I had. He said I could be given a local anaesthetic, and the vocal cords could be accessed from the outside (causing yet another scar on my neck). My jaw joint was too weak for him to access the cords from the back of the throat, as I could not open my mouth wide enough since having the meniscectomy back in November 2006. I could just imagine lying on the operating table wide awake whilst my neck was being sliced open for the third time (why not put a zip in the damn thing!). He stressed that I had to be awake so that I could talk to him and he could hear if my voice was improving as he was working away. Hmm…I would have to think about that one. I had a mental picture of me trying to climb off the operating table in mid-procedure. What with the dacryocystorhinostomies possibly on the cards, the operations were backing up again.

My eyes stayed clear and dry for the rest of May without any treatment at all. I was cautiously beginning to think I wouldn't have any more problems. This was put to the test however, when Phil and I had a day at Great Yarmouth with our youngest son Matt and his fiancé Anna at the end of May. For those who have never been to

Yarmouth, there is usually a chilly East wind that blows for most of the year, and this was unfortunately quite prevalent on our day trip. My eyes started watering almost as soon as I got out of the car, and continued to do so for the rest of the day. Things went from bad to worse, and during the following week I was plagued with an infection in my left eye that would not go away. Remembering that the ophthalmologist wanted to see me when the infection was active, I telephoned his secretary only to be told that he was on holiday and would be back the following week. I made an appointment for 2nd June, knowing that I couldn't treat the infection at all as he wanted to see my eyes in their worst state. The waiting to be seen was quite, quite miserable, and so was I.

The ophthalmologist noticed quite a bit of stickiness around my left eye, and said rather than keep prescribing strong steroids (which was not a good idea as they could eventually cause cataracts) and antibiotics, he needed to find a reason for the constant infections. He asked if I would be amenable to a 'tear duct washout'. When I asked if that required a hospital stay, he said not at all and that he could do it there and then. The procedure might be a bit 'uncomfortable' (the medical profession always understate this word), but would let him know if the tear duct was blocked or not. I agreed to him carrying out this procedure, and so he placed some anaesthetic drops in my left eye and drew up some sterile fluid in a syringe. He injected this into the left tear duct, and said that if the duct worked normally I would soon taste the fluid in the back of my throat. Unfortunately I did not, and the fluid shot back out down my cheek instead of going down my throat. This indeed showed that the tear duct was blocked and was the reason for all my problems. I had known all along it was not the blepharitis I had previously been told I had by the GP and by the eye clinic at the hospital where I worked. At last we had a diagnosis.

The ophthalmologist said that unblocking tear ducts would probably require surgery, and this was not his speciality. He would refer me to an eye surgeon who did these operations all the time (dacryocystorhinostomies). Another consultant (I've lost count now of how many I have seen)! I made an appointment on the way out to see the new eye surgeon the following week, who also worked at the Cambridge Lea hospital. The ophthalmologist also prescribed some Chloramphenicol antibiotic eye drops, which cleared the symptoms up in a few days.

I still had no symptoms when the new eye surgeon syringed both tear ducts again the following week. The left eye was still partly blocked even though I had no symptoms, but the right eye seemed fine. He said I would need an operation to unblock the left naso-lacrimal duct, or else the infections would get worse and worse. This would take about 45 minutes under a general anaesthetic, and I would be left with some bruising and swelling afterwards which would take about a fortnight to go. The operation had a 95% success rate. After the operation I would have some stitches in and a stent, and both would require removal – the stitches about a week after surgery, and the stent after about six weeks. There would be no hot drinks for two days following surgery, and no nose-blowing for a week as both could set off nosebleeds. He was not going to approach the duct via the nostril, as I had a deviated septum and there was not enough room for him to get all his toolkit in there. He would access the duct from the outside, and I would have a small scar at the top of my nose that would not be noticeable as I wore glasses which would cover it up. What's another scar? I have a huge one on my neck, so the more the merrier! He had the date of 14th July 2009 free. The operation would be performed about 5pm. He did not think the right side needed any treatment, and said that once the blockage was treated, the right side would probably clear up by itself.

The wife of Phil's boss was very helpful. She put me in touch with a friend of hers, Linda, who had had radiation for breast cancer, and also had suffered from watery infected eyes afterwards (it's amazing the Eye Clinic where I work did not make this connection - they must see thousands of people a year) and had undergone the same operation as I was going to have. Linda said her operation was a success for two years, but she was now suffering the watery eyes again and was thinking about getting the procedure done a second time. I did not realise the problem could come back. The eye surgeon had told me that accessing the duct from the outside instead of via the nostril was the 'Gold Standard' to work by, and this way the problem did not recur, so I was ever hopeful mine would be a lasting success.

CHAPTER 30 – DOWNLOAD FESTIVAL

Meanwhile there was the Download music festival to enjoy whilst waiting for 14th July to come around. The festival was held at Donnington Park racecourse in the Midlands. The night before I came down with a nasty bout of cystitis and wondered if I would be able to go at all. The GP surgery as usual had no appointments for that day, so I looked in our medicine cabinet and found some very strong antibiotics, Ciprofloxacin, which had been given to me three years' previously in Addenbrooke's whilst undergoing radiation treatment. This cleared up the problem almost immediately, and I looked forward to the festival.

It was with some degree of heartsink when we were met on arrival at the West car park by possibly the same very amiable but charmingly persistent nun collecting money for her cause, who had also accosted us at the Isle of Wight festival the year before. Extracting ourselves from her clutches and two pounds lighter already, we asked directions to the campsite from one of the many 'car park police' dotted about. He pointed a finger and said it was 'that way up the hill'.

'Up the hill' turned out to be an hour's trudge to the family camping site lugging the last of the camping gear. Luckily Phil and Matt had set up the tents the day before, in order to bag a good spot not too far away from the festibogs (but not too near either). Matt had returned home as he and Anna were attending the May ball at Anna's college the next evening (they would return on Saturday), and Phil had returned home to collect the last of the gear and our eldest son Lee and I after we had finished work the following day.

The family camping site was described as a place for 'people who want to enjoy the festival, but who also would like some peace and quiet'. It cost us a few pounds more for the privilege, but that suited us nicely. I looked forward to this island of calm and stillness in the midst of the usual racket of alcoholic and debauched festivity going on all around. Phil had mentioned that the previous night when he stayed in the tent, there seemed to be quite a few aeroplanes flying overhead.

Yes, there were. He was right. Somebody in their wisdom on the website failed to mention that the whole Download site was under one of the main flight paths out of the East Midlands airport, a stone's throw away. As we settled into our tent, every few minutes another plane came roaring over our heads, taking passengers away from the aforesaid alcoholic and debauched festivity going on below. Also, the family camping site was a short walk from the fairground rides that entertained 75,000 people into the small hours after the main arena closed. Peace and quiet? You must be joking!

Time to check out the loos. The festibogs were humming nicely in the mid-afternoon sun and pollulating with festeringness. An alarming festibug could gain entry to your unsuspecting digestive system with ease with only one visit to these gruesome establishments.

Nevertheless we were all set to enjoy the festival. Phil started pumping up the airbeds, and I looked around for my bag of clothes to find a pair of long trousers to change into, as it had suddenly become a tad chilly. It then hit me with a sickening thud that said bag of clothes and toiletries were still sitting at the top of our stairs ready to be packed into the car. I had not brought them downstairs, and neither had Phil. Lee looked as though he wanted to be somewhere else, as he sensed a domestic brewing. It just gets better and better doesn't it! Lee suggested buying some more clothes, but Phil kindly offered to go back and get them. I did not want to waste money on buying unnecessary clothing, so we made the decision to go back home after Motley Crue had played that evening, stay at home for the night, and then return with the bag of contention the next day. Lee would stay behind and meet up that night with some old workmates that were also attending the festival.

It was time to walk to the arena to see the bands play. It was possibly a half hour's walk from the campsite to the arena, and we were joined on our travels by a few thousand new arrivals eager to check out the sounds. Young people seemed to outnumber us middle-agers by about 10:1. We came to the conclusion our peers either did not like the music, could not do the walking, did not like camping, or maybe it was a combination of all three. The Isle of Wight festival seemed to attract many more middle-agers, but then there was a bit less walking there, and the music was less death-orientated. Perhaps we're just unusual in liking heavy metal!

By the time we arrived at the arena at about 7pm, Limp Bizkit were just finishing their set on the main stage and Korn were starting theirs. Lee wandered off to meet up with his friends and watch Korn. Not being a fan of either band we were not too bothered – we preferred to watch Opeth and Motley Crue play on the second stage. We said our goodbyes to Lee as we wouldn't see him until the next day.

Back at the South car park on the Saturday, we looked out for the nun but she wasn't there – she probably had had to go to the bank with a wheelbarrow to deposit her takings. Matt and Anna were arriving soon. I gave Matt a ring to find out where he was. After quite a while a sleepy voice answered. They had slept through the alarm after partying hard at the May ball. He'd missed his chance to see Ripper Owens at 11am, and it would be some time before they saw any bands at all. We left the bag in the car, as we had previously booked a Travelodge room some months back for the middle night to have a bath and a good night's sleep, being the sensible people that we were. I had not actually slept in the tent yet, but hey, I could not resist the pull of the bath and a bed over an airbed and a tent.

We arrived back at the arena just in time to witness the 'awesome' Five Finger Death Punch on the main stage. The poor singer was angry at the world and hated everybody, even himself. Nobody loved him, he knew. After a warning to the more timid front-of-stagers to move back, he then got on with a song which I think was called 'I'm taking it back with my knuckles'. This involved the entire mosh pit at the front punching each other senseless (if they weren't already with the influence of several Jagermeisters) and shouting the aforementioned song title at the same time. The audience loved it, and the medical centre at the back of the arena was on standby. It was awesome to watch.

Not only did I not want to be in the front-of –stage moshpit, I actually did not want to be at the front at all. There was an unearthly pong all around the front of the stage area. People who were 'lucky' enough to get a spot stayed there all day. If they needed the loo, I think they did it there and then judging by the smell, which was coupled with the stench of stale beer and body odour. Beer bottles were used as receptacles for urine which were then tossed into the crowd. Am I making it sound agreeable enough for you? Phil and I agreed it was much better to sit nearer the back. You could still hear everything just as well as if you were at the front, but you were less likely to get hit by a bottle of urine.

My favourite band of the day were The Answer, who we had also seen at the Isle of Wight festival the year before. They followed Static-X, another good band, and were due to play at 4.25pm on the second stage. We had met up with Matt, Anna, and Lee by this time, and we all got as near to the front as we could (without being knocked out by the smell), as I'd previously told them about The Answer and they were all keen to see them. Lee and Matt were wearing tutus, but nobody took any notice. Anything went at Download. Two steel barriers a few feet apart separated us from the VIP's right at the front of the stage who had paid twice the amount for their tickets. This chasm was supervised by the 'arena police' who stood with their backs to the stage watching us, in case anybody dared to vault the barriers and join the VIP's.

The Answer are from Belfast and had obviously grown up listening to Led Zeppelin's music. The singer even looks like Robert Plant with his long blonde hair. However, their songs are their own. Matt picked up their influences straight away, and Lee, Matt and Anna rocked away until it was time for them to run round to the main stage to see Pendulum, then run back to the second stage to see The Prodigy (they had some unwanted attention in their tutus in the Prodigy's mosh pit), and then they would hopefully get back to the main stage in time to catch the last of Slipknot's set. Before Slipknot we managed to meet up again and catch Thunder's set on the Tuborg stage. Unfortunately Thunder were to be no more after Download, so we made the most of it, singing along to 'Love Walked In' and their version of 'Gimme Some Lovin' amongst many others. Saturday night was also our chance to live in the lap of luxury at the Travelodge. The next night it would be the tent for me, and the festibogs.

Sunday was the best day as far as I was concerned. Phil took our overnight bags from the car back to the tent before all the best bands started on the main stage about 2.30pm. The 'campsite police' searched in my bag (yes, the bag of contention) and found a strange metal object which they wanted Phil to take out for their inspection. To his embarrassment it was my hairdryer (Travelodge's have electricity!). Now why was this man taking a hairdryer to a tent? Phil did not have an answer either, and cursed the ****ing bag under his breath all over again. The 'campsite police' let it through, as there was no way he could use it for anything!

Just look at this lineup on Sunday afternoon; 2.30 Journey, 3.35 Dream Theater, 3.55 ZZ Top (are those beards real?), 6.35 Whitesnake, and to top it all at 8.45 there was Def Leppard to headline. I was in rock heaven and so was everybody else. I particularly remember hearing the audience erupt as Dream Theater came on stage and went straight into 'Pull Me Under'. Yes. It was worth sleeping in a tent for this. Anna had to return home on Sunday evening due to work commitments, so it was decided that I would sleep in Matt and Anna's small tent, and the three boys would share the big tent. I did not fancy sharing a tent with three blokes who had been on the beer all day (you know – winds moderate to gusting /disgusting and all that…)

On the way back to the campsite at the end of the festival, we passed the 'Comfy Crappers'. We had passed them on the Friday and Saturday, but now seemed the right time to check them out as the festibogs had started making Matt and I retch. Lee was using a nearby tree /fence, and Phil just wanted to wait until he got home before doing anything at all. The blokes all seemed to be using the fence opposite our tent for a wee, and Anna had been quite dismayed on joining the early Sunday morning festibog queue to be last after 30 blokes, each holding a loo roll. She returned to the tent announcing she would 'wait a while longer'!

There was a bit of a queue for the Comfy Crappers, but not too bad. Phil and I joined the queue whilst the boys went back to the tent. The Crappers are composting toilets and do not smell. I was all for that. Each person in the queue paid £2.50 and was given a wooden spoon. You can imagine the conversation Phil and I were having as to the purpose of this instrument. I came up with the idea that as the loos were composted, then once you had done your business you dug some earth out of a well-placed bucket and covered your traces. Phil's brain raced away and his ideas are probably best left unsaid.

For my £2.50 I expected a virtual state-of –the- art flushing toilet. What I got differed wildly from what I had imagined. The long handle of the wooden spoon was used to put into two holes in the door to 'lock' it, and there was a wooden box with a hole in it on which you sat to do your business. Granted you had loo paper, but that was it. At least there was no pong to the loos though, but I wouldn't actually say they were 'comfy'. You were given some hand sanitizer on exiting.

Now then, I could not put it off any more. It was time to sleep in Matt and Anna's pygmy tent. How they both managed to get any sleep in it baffled me terribly. Phil had put one of our airbeds in it for me, and the higher end of the airbed was facing me as I unzipped the tent. I crawled over it and tried to make myself comfortable. A plane went overhead. Snoring came from our neighbours on either side. The fairground was in full swing. Rain pitter-patted on the plastic outer cover. I wanted my Travelodge room. I was still in my clothes because I knew I would need the festibogs again sometime during the night. Another plane went overhead. This sucked already and I had only been laying there for 10 minutes.

I must have dozed off eventually about 4am, and was woken at 5.30 by our neighbours packing up to go home. This seemed to wake up the rest of the campsite, and most people were up and packing up by 6.30. A plane went overhead. The 'tent police' patrolled and made sure everyone was awake. Another plane took off. One tent was still upright with no sign of life. The 'tent police' unzipped the cover and looked inside. Had somebody died of alcoholic poisoning overnight? The tent was unoccupied so they started to take it down. The poor owner might have gone to the festibogs and wanted a Monday morning lie-in afterwards! No such luck. It was pack up and go home time. A plane went by overhead. We had rocked 'till we dropped.

Throughout this debauchery I had had no eye symptoms whatsoever. It was just my luck that now the operation was booked, the eye problem would spontaneously resolve by itself.

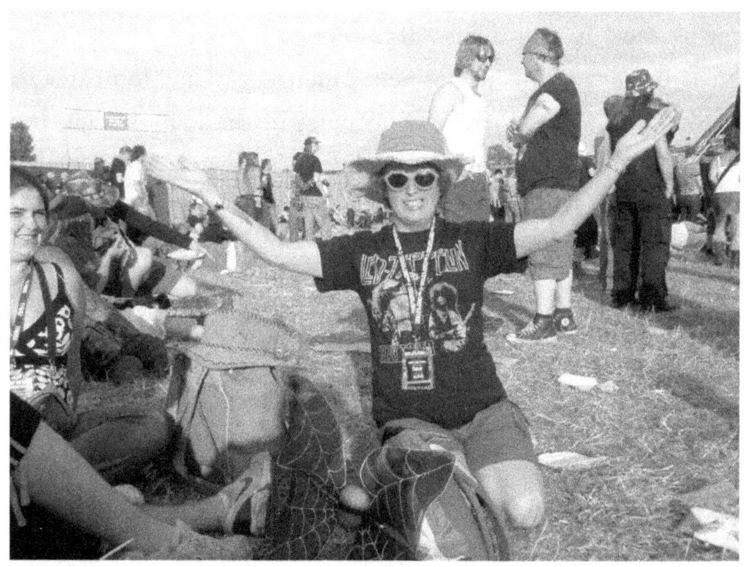

Photo shows Anna and I at Download June 2009.

CHAPTER 31 – LEFT EYE DACRYOCYSTORHINOSTOMY

Over the next few weeks I did not get as many symptoms as before, but enough watering of the left eye to know that I still needed the operation. We had had a week's annual leave in early July and visited Althorp, Princess Diana's childhood home, and attended an Eagles' concert in Birmingham's National Indoor Arena. The weather had not been too great, and walking around outside in the cold wind usually started the watering eye symptoms off. I viewed the day of the operation with mixed feelings; relief to finally have two normal dry eyes at last, but dismay at having to undergo yet another general anaesthetic.

I was not due in Theatre until 4pm, so did not have to arrive at the hospital until 3.15pm. It's much better sitting at home than in the hospital all day, especially as I suffer from 'white coat syndrome' every time (as soon as they come round with the observation machine my blood pressure and pulse rise automatically). I was able to have my usual bowl of porridge at 06.45 but nothing more to eat after that, although I was able to carry on sipping water until 10am.

When we arrived at the Spire Lea hospital I was shown to my room. The hospital is all on the ground floor. Room 107 was quite small, but had its own bathroom and toilet facilities. I ordered a light supper for later on after the operation, and then was visited by the surgeon and anaesthetist after being admitted by the nurse in charge. The surgeon took my consent and as they usually do, letting me know all the side-effects the operation might consist of; these being bleeding from the nose, and a bruised and swollen face for a couple of weeks afterwards. He did say the operation had about a 95% success rate, so I was quite happy to sign the consent form. I told the anaesthetist of the phlegm problem at the back of my throat I had had for three years (also caused by the radiation I had), and he said it would not be a problem. It was then time for me to get into my gown and be taken to Theatre.

Phil walked down to Theatre with me, but was not allowed to go into the anaesthetic room. Into the cannula in my arm went the liquid cosh. I was told I would feel like I had had a couple too many gins. I started to tell them I didn't like gin, but didn't remember any more until somebody in the Recovery room was asking me to 'open my eye'. It was all over. My left eye had a large white patch over it; hence I was only able to open one eye, not both. I was desperate for a sip of water and asked the Recovery nurse for a drink. I was told to only sip a few mouthfuls as it was too soon after the operation to take a lot of liquid in. The water tasted like manna!

After about a half hour in Recovery, I was wheeled back to my room where dear Phil was waiting for me. There was a blood pressure cuff attached to my right arm, and this inflated at regular intervals. As usual my blood pressure and pulse were high, as my body does not like anaesthetics. Phil gave me small sips of water, and I slowly woke up. The surgeon and anaesthetist came in to see me, and were pleased with the outcome of the operation. I had small incision on the left side of my nose with a couple of stitches in, and there was a stent keeping the new drainage channel open. The surgeon said if I wanted to go home then I could go that evening if I felt well enough. I knew I would have some reaction to the anaesthetic and did not fancy going home that evening.

After about four hours I managed to eat a small chicken sandwich, but felt dreadfully sick afterwards. Phil called the nurse and she administered an anti-sickness drug through the cannula that worked quite quickly and made me feel better within about 10 minutes. Following this, the evening nursing staff made it quite clear that Phil was not allowed to stay in my room all night, and that he had to go home. He had been such a help to me and had saved the nurses work, so we could not work out why they wanted him out. He left about midnight.

It was during the night that another reaction to the anaesthetic kicked in. Again I suffered an over-production of thick phlegm running down the back of the nose. I could not shift it and thought at one point it was going to get stuck in my windpipe. This always happens to me after operations, and I knew I would need a couple of nebulisers to help loosen the phlegm. I mentioned the problem to the morning nursing staff, and the emergency doctor was called in to listen to my chest. I tried to explain that the phlegm was originally a by-product of the radioiodine treatment I had three years previously. It is always there in a mild form, and it does not come up from my lungs but goes down the back of my nose and into my throat. Colds and operations make the phlegm problem worse. The doctor was not listening, listened to my chest, and said my chest was clear (I could have told him that). However, he did prescribe a nebuliser after I told him it does help after operations. The physiotherapist heard the nebuliser going, came in and said she wanted to listen to my chest. I gave up trying to explain my problem and let her get on with it. She also said my chest was clear!

After a couple of nebulisers I felt a bit better and was able to go home. The nurse took the eye patch off and put some small steri-strips on the wound, so I was able to wear my glasses. I had to come back nine days later for the stitches to be taken out, but the stenting tube was not going to be taken out until August 27th. I was not allowed to have any hot drinks for two days and could not blow my nose for a week, in case of setting off nosebleeds. I was given an eye patch to wear at night to stop me scratching my eye (it was already itchy), and some Maxitrol eye drops to be taken four times a day for a month (a steroid to stop infections). I was also not allowed to do any strenuous activity for three weeks afterwards, again because of the risk of setting off nosebleeds. I had booked two weeks off work as sick leave, but now it looked as if I would need three weeks. After collecting my discharge letter from the main desk to give to my GP, I was allowed to go home.

It took quite a few days to recover from the anaesthetic. On the first day home I felt quite shaky and could not eat much. Bruising and swelling came out over my left eye and cheekbone, and I looked as if I had been in the boxing ring for a few rounds. On the fourth day I felt well enough to attend my granddaughter Sophie's fourth birthday party. The bruising was receding a bit, and with sunglasses on I hoped I would not frighten all the little partygoers! It took roughly a week for me to feel back to normal, and I went back to work after two weeks and back to the gym after three weeks. I was lucky not to suffer any nosebleeds at all. The only thing I noticed was that the stenting tube still caused my left eye to water a bit, as the tears could not drain properly with the tube in the way, but other than that and the bruising, there was no actual pain, just a bit of tenderness around the site of the incision. Also I could just about see the tiny stenting tube in the corner of my eye. My left eye looked smaller than the right while the tubes were in, and to the uninitiated it looked like I had no corner to my eye at all.

On August 27th, nearly six weeks after the operation, I visited the surgeon again to have the stenting tubes out. First of all he asked me to blow my nose and for the air to come out of the left nostril, as that would cause the tubes to come lower down in the nostril. He then cut the stenting tube in the corner of my eye, and then tried to get the tubes out by pulling them out of my nostril. It was becoming decidedly uncomfortable for me whilst he was trying to do this, so he gave me a local anaesthetic spray in the nostril which helped a bit. He said there was not much room in the left nostril in which to work, and I wondered if the tubes were stuck up there for good. Finally with a lot of tugging they came out, but I felt decidedly shaky afterwards and just sat still for a while. The surgeon said to make another appointment with him in three months' time for the last check-up. Apparently it would be ok for me to cancel it if I felt I did not need it.

Thank goodness for that. It was all over. The watery eyes cleared up wonderfully once the stenting tubes were taken out, and on 6th September it was time to forget about it all and head for a well-earned holiday in the Isle of Wight.

We had a great week's holiday. The sun shone, and it was very warm for the time of year. We visited the old favourites; the Needles (by chairlift and boat), Puckpool beach, Ryde, Ventnor (rather scary ghost walk at night around the botanical gardens), and Tennyson's house at Freshwater (now the Farringford hotel). There was a nasty moment a few days before we left to get the ferry, when my left eye became pus-filled for a day, although there was no watering. I applied some more Maxitrol drops and the eye cleared up the same day, whereas before it would have taken about three or four days. I had no trouble with either eye whilst we were away, and I tenuously held out hope that the eye infections were a thing of the past.

They seemed to be. September, October and November came and went and my eyes seemed as normal as everybody else's. I was so pleased to be cured of the constant infections. I cancelled my check-up appointment with the eye surgeon at the end of November, because as far as I was concerned, I did not need it any more. All I needed sometimes were liquid tear drops at night, as after a few hours' sleep my eyes often felt dry, but that was the only problem I had. I could even walk outside in a howling gale and my eyes did not water. The miracle of surgery!

CHAPTER 32 - MRI SCAN AND CHECK-UP

As the end of the year approached, it was time for another scan of my neck and a check –up with my oncologist. This time I had to have an MRI (magnetic resonance imaging) scan, as too many CT scans over the years would give me an accumulation of too much radiation, possibly causing leukaemia. At work I had seen many MRI request forms returned to us, as the patient was 'too claustrophobic' to enter the scanner. This had indeed put the wind up me, and I imagined being enclosed in a tunnel for half an hour quietly going demented listening to the noise of the scanner and wondering if everybody had forgotten about me. I asked Phil if he would mind coming in the room with me. I felt I could probably tolerate it if I knew he was there, as he would not forget I was in there! Of course he agreed, and I phoned the MRI nurse to make sure his presence would not be a problem. She assured me that Phil would be welcome in the room, and I relaxed a bit.

On entering the MRI suite we were both asked to take off any metal, so off came my earrings, wedding ring and watch, and off came Phil's belt and wedding ring. We were asked if we had any metalwork in our bodies, and were allowed to enter the scanner room when we replied in the negative. I could see the scanner was not an enclosed tunnel, but was open at the back. What a relief! I then had to lie on my back on the entrance to the scanner, and my head was encased in a vice ensuring I couldn't move it. I was given earplugs to put in my ears, as a magnetic scanner is very noisy, and then I was moved inside the scanner. I closed my eyes so that I wouldn't feel enclosed and claustrophobic, and Phil could just about reach my right hand to hold it, which felt very reassuring. Then came 20 minutes of loud noises as the scanner did its thing. I was given a contrast injection halfway through, to enhance the pictures for viewing, and was then allowed to go home to await the results on December 7th. I hoped I was still in remission.

Whilst waiting for the results, something quite unexpected happened. I was asked to help co-run the UK branch of the Bon Jovi fan club! In his line of work, Phil often had cause to visit one of the Cambridge universities, and over the years had forged a good working relationship with Helen, one of the technicians there. One day on visiting Helen, he noticed that she was wearing a festival wristband. He mentioned that we also often attended music festivals, and the whole thing mushroomed from there. At first Helen told Phil that her brother was able to obtain VIP tickets for festivals through his work. She promised to get us some VIP tickets to the Download 2010 and Sonisphere festivals, and then she mentioned she was at the last Bon Jovi concert at Twickenham, sitting on the side of the stage (VIP ticket again!). Phil and I were also at the Twickenham concert (sitting at the back of the stadium though), and Helen mentioned that she used to run the Bon Jovi fan club in the nineties, so was still getting VIP tickets from the band. She said she could get us a framed, signed photo of the band, and that she was thinking of starting up the fan club again.

True to her word, the next time Phil visited Helen's workplace she had the framed photo for us, which the band had signed, and by this time Helen and I were in regular email contact, although had not met. Helen asked Phil if I would be interested in helping her run the fan club, and we all arranged to meet to discuss it.

Matt turned 24 in the two weeks in-between the scan and the results. Celebrations seemed to go on for about three days. At one point Matt and several of the male birthday party guests/ soon to be wedding guests decided to look for their wedding suits and visited Newmarket High Street to choose the suits they were going to hire.

At last it was the day for getting the MRI results. As usual my heart was beating extra fast with nerves as I went into the consultant's surgery. Did I need another operation on my neck to remove any more nodes? The consultant again was all smiles as she had been the previous year; my MRI looked good, and there were no problems. All I needed was a blood test to check my thyroxine level, and a bone scan to check for osteoporosis (as being over-medicated on thyroxine could possibly cause this). I would see her again in a year's time. I heaved a sigh of relief. Now it was time to enjoy the lead up to Christmas.

Lee and Sarah came to visit on Christmas Eve with the girls, and we all sat down to dinner together. We would not be seeing them on Christmas Day as they were spending it with Sarah's parents, so we made the most of it and opened all our presents. Sophie especially was thrilled with her karaoke machine, and gave impromptu performances throughout the evening.

Christmas Day was spent with my mother and Matt and Anna at Anna's parents' house. Alison provided a lovely dinner as always, and there were more presents to open after dinner. We also returned on New Year's Eve to attend their party. Fireworks heralded the start of 2010 in their garden at midnight.

CHAPTER 33 - BONE SCAN AND RESULTS OF BLOOD TESTS.

There was heavy snow during the first week of January 2010. Phil and I met up with Helen, who confirmed we would now be running the Bon Jovi fan club for the whole of Europe, which was rather daunting. Mostly though it seemed to involve answering queries by email and forwarding details of merchandise orders to the distribution depot. There was to be a meeting with Jon Bon Jovi himself in London in June to go over the details. Helen had also given Jon Bon Jovi himself a CD of Aeon Zen, the band that Matt played guitar in, and Jon was much impressed and predicted a bright future for them. There was much to look forward to in 2010, especially the Download, Sonisphere, and High Voltage festivals, and of course Matt and Anna's wedding.

The results of my thyroid function blood test came through in mid-January; The anti-thyroglobulin antibodies had reduced even further to 310 (I think they were about 1000 before I was in remission), but my thyroid stimulating hormone (TSH) level was not low enough to achieve full suppression (probably because I had put on a little weight and was more active in the gym), so I had to increase my thyroxine to 175mg three times a week and 150mg four times a week to try and keep the TSH under 0.03. Another blood test after eight weeks confirmed thyroxine levels were correct.

Also Soon after Christmas came the summons to attend for a bone scan at the Nuffield hospital in Bury. This one was not as bad as the MRI; it was not enclosed, and I just had to lie flat while the scanner took some images of my spine and left hip. The result was that I had a normal bone density for my age, and I only had a 0.2% chance of a fracture of the hip and a 4% chance of a fracture anywhere else. Another one would not be due for at least 4 – 6 years.

I had stopped taking the norethisterone tablets in December, as my periods were getting very much lighter and I assumed the menopause was imminent. It seemed as soon as I had stopped taking them the menopause kicked in with the start of the dreaded hot flushes. At first I was not sure whether it was the increased thyroxine or the menopause causing the flushes, but a blood test in February confirmed my FSH and LH hormones were high (indicating I was menopausal). A work colleague suggested sage as an alternative to HRT, as it was well-known in reducing the amount of hot flushes. I started taking capsules consisting of a combination of herbs and 50% sage, and waited hopefully for a result. After a month or so I was still getting flushes, but not so many. The sage seemed to be making a slight difference. I decided to just take the norethisterone tablets for 8 days only when I started getting PMT symptoms. Hopefully if my periods were on the wane, then I would not be getting so many.

An old condition, tennis elbows, flared up again in the early part of February. I had had this condition since working as a ward clerk in 2002, but now I suppose the constant typing I did and the gripping of medical notes made it worse. The consultant I worked for injected some steroid and local anaesthetic into both elbows which seemed to settle it down somewhat.

Preparations for Matt and Anna's wedding got underway properly in Spring. I visited a dressmaker recommended by Anna's mother who was going to make me a silk and lace dress for the wedding. I was quite excited that I would actually have a dress that fitted me, as I was quite a peculiar shape; having no waist meant that a dress bought to fit the hips and bust was too small around the waist, and a dress that fitted the waist was too big around the bust and hips. We visited the reception venue and went over the details with the Wedding Planner. All was set for August 6th.

A disaster occurred in April. Lee and Sarah's house was damaged by fire. The fire started in the door of their dishwasher, which was on standby at the time and not even on. Luckily nobody was in the house at the time, but the fire smouldered for three hours and the whole house was covered in black smoke and soot. They lost everything and were only left with the clothes they stood up in. They were insured thank goodness, but had to move out to a rented house whilst repairs were made. Their insurance company were wonderful; they gave them an emergency cheque straight away for £2000 to cover immediate expenses, paid the rent on a house nearby for them, and organised builders to repair the damage. All together Lee and Sarah were in the rented house for four months, but at the end of it they moved back into a completely renovated refurbished house all paid for by CIS Insurance.

Another six-month check-up was due with the ENT surgeon in May. I had been getting symptoms of a 'catch' or tickle in the back of my throat since Christmas, although by the appointment in May the symptoms seemed to be resolving somewhat. This tickle would make my eyes and nose run and sometimes make me sneeze. I was getting many of these per day, and wondered what it was. The ENT surgeon looked down the back of my throat via a camera through the nostril, and announced everything looked normal. He felt all around my neck but could find nothing wrong (a few years later I realised it was hormonal, as it cleared up in 2014 with the menopause in full swing). Another clear check –up then, and another appointment for a year's time. He would liaise with the oncologist to decide whether I needed another MRI scan this year.

The sage and anti-inflammatory food supplements I was taking made me feel so good and so free of knee pain that I started running again at weekends. I had changed my diet to cut out carbohydrates, and felt a lot more alert. I wanted to lose some weight for the wedding, and embarked on a no/low carbohydrate diet. I cut out potatoes rice, bread and pasta, and lost four pounds in the first two weeks. Phil and I ran/walked four miles every weekend, and I visited the gym twice or three times a week. The weight loss slowed down after the first month, but I definitely felt a lot more alert. I wanted to combine my cancer-free state with healthy living and try and make my body heal itself.

Unfortunately nothing seemed to stop the catches in my throat or the hot flushes. I did not want to take HRT because of the risk of breast cancer – I would probably get that as well I thought. It would just be my luck. I had to grin and bear both of these symptoms; my face would flush a pillar-box red many times during the day, and I was forever coughing as the catch would attack the back of my throat and make me want to retch.

Over a period of time I realised that the throat catches and hot flushes were cyclical in nature. When I was taking norethisterone for PMT symptoms, the catches and flushes were absent. I read on the internet that norethisterone is a muscle relaxant, and so I assumed it relaxed the muscles in the back of my throat. When I stopped taking the norethisterone I knew I'd have a period 2 days later, and when this was over the flushes and catches started again until the PMT returned. Sometimes it would be 6 weeks before I needed to take any more tablets, sometimes only three weeks, and sometimes more than two months.

During May was the first of the hen parties. A group of Anna's friends, her sister-in-law Laura (who was heavily pregnant, hence the reason for the first party so that Laura could take part!), Anna's Mum Alison and I all went to London for the day for shopping, lunch, and then to see a show, Legally Blonde, in The Strand. Alison booked a stretch limo for the day, and we travelled in style, turning heads as we got out of the limo at Covent Garden. Lunch was at the very 'unusual' restaurant 'Saracens' in Covent Garden (anybody ever been in the toilets there.....!) frequented I think by many famous thespians.

The famous meeting in June to discuss running the fan club with Bon Jovi unfortunately failed to materialise. Reading between the lines I got the impression from Helen that somebody else had been given the job. It was a great disappointment to me, but decided at the end of the day that I could do nothing to change the situation, so stopped worrying about it. Communication with Helen dwindled to nothing after a few months, and I drew a line under the whole affair.

However, there were other things to look forward to in June. Phil, Lee, Matt, Anna and I all took our tents and camped at the Download festival again. Helen had given us VIP guest passes some weeks previously, and this year we had access to the VIP area where we used to meet up after each band had finished playing. There was shelter there if it rained, a bar, BBQ, and toilets of a much higher calibre (which is always a good thing!). We enjoyed the likes of AC/DC, Saxon, Cinderella, Megadeth and Motorhead. The weather stayed fine until just before Aerosmith were due to play, and then it absolutely bucketed down gnd the whole site turned into a mudbath. It was like Woodstock all over again. At that point lots of people went home, but we hadn't taken the tents down that morning, so we trudged back to the tent in the mud and stayed another night listening to the rain hammering on the canvas.

The heat returned for another concert in June – this time to see Pearl Jam in Hyde Park. We roasted in the heat that day along with several thousand other people all sitting on the grass enjoying the music.

July was the start of the wedding celebrations in earnest after rocking at the High Voltage and Sonisphere festivals. There was a second hen night at Newmarket races (I won £18.50!), and a stag weekend in Amsterdam. I think all the boys returned a bit the worse for wear, but on the whole according to Phil it was a 'civilised' stag do (is there such a thing?). There was wedding shower for Anna a few nights before the wedding, and a rehearsal and family dinner the night before. The pre-wedding celebrations had stretched out over a month or so, and finally the big day arrived.

Matt stayed with us the night before the wedding. Unfortunately he and Phil had to be up early on the wedding morning and travel to the reception in order to set the music system up (they could not gain access to the reception venue the day before as another wedding was taking place). I told them to take their hired suits with them in case there was a hold up on the A12 and they ran out of time to get to the church. Fortunately they arrived back just as I was returning from the hairdressers, so we all travelled together to St. Margaret's Church in Ipswich, where Matt and Anna were married in the most beautiful wedding ceremony I had ever seen. Anna's friends from her choir sang an amazing version of 'Jesu Joy of Man's Desiring' as she walked down the aisle with her father. There was so much love in the church for that young couple that you could almost touch it. I was even crying at the wedding rehearsal and thought I would need a wheelbarrow –load of tissues on the day itself, but they looked so happy and so in love that I was happy for them and smiled all the way through the service instead!

The reception was held at Le Talbooth at Dedham. A marquee had been erected in the grounds, and about 80 people sat down to a superb buffet, and danced the night away to music that Matt had prepared himself beforehand. The happy couple honeymooned in Toronto, staying in a cottage owned by a relative of Anna's mother.

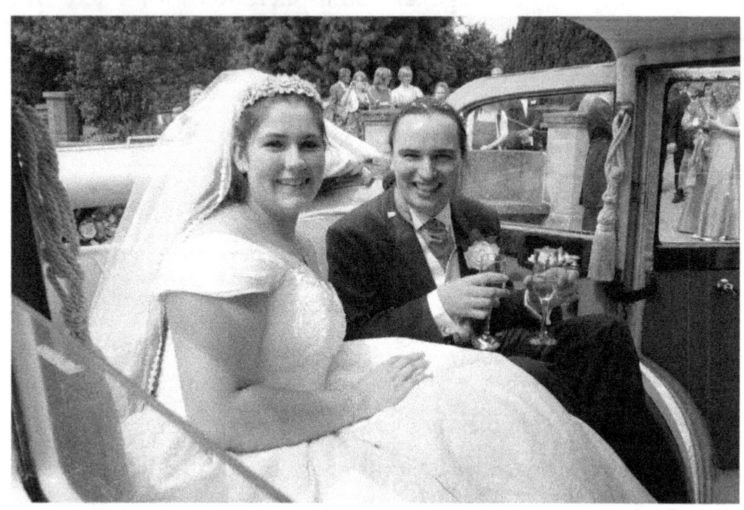

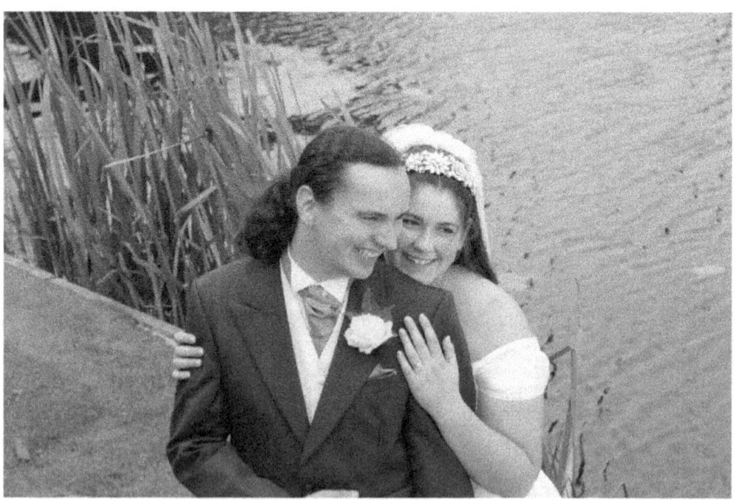

CHAPTER 34 – A PAIN
IN THE ELBOWS

Soon after the wedding the tennis elbow condition flared up again in earnest. The pain was constant and unremitting. The consultant I worked for said it was not a good idea to have too many steroid injections, and referred me for nerve conduction studies at the Norfolk & Norwich hospital (I was diagnosed with carpal tunnel syndrome). I visited the GP who referred me for some physio, referred me to an orthopaedic surgeon, and signed me off work for a month. I hoped that if I had a rest from the constant typing it might settle the symptoms down again and I would not need surgery, but unfortunately neither the rest, a holiday in the Isle of Wight in early September, physiotherapy, or eventually reduced working hours were successful. Because I had had the condition on and off for about 8 years, the orthopaedic surgeon said nothing probably would work except surgery. He could perform a tennis elbow release procedure for me under local anaesthetic (what a relief – no after-effects of a general!). I had hoped 2010 would be the year of no operations at all, but it was not to be as the procedure on the left arm was now booked for November 11ᵗʰ. When that arm had healed then the right elbow would be operated on, and I would be off work for about four months in all. As November approached I even began to look forward to the operation on the left elbow, as the pain had progressed up to the bicep muscle in that arm and also the shoulder, and both arms were stiff and sore.

However, come November 11th I was struck down with a rather nasty cold and the operation had to be postponed to January 13th. I had actually gone through 2010 with no operations after all! I think fate had intervened though, because on November 10th my mother had had to suddenly move out of her sheltered accommodation due to a heating oil leak, and move into the guest room of a sheltered housing unit near to our home. She lived there for two months before another flat became available, and during that time we helped her relocate and move into another flat, finally finishing and ensuring she was self-sufficient on January 12th, the day before the postponed operation. I could never have helped her with one arm in a cast!

Towards the end of November I acted upon the advice of a friend whose hot flushes had been successfully treated with homeopathy. The sage capsules had not really worked in reducing them for me, and I did not want to start on HRT due to the risk of breast cancer. My friend gave me the name (Debbie) and number of the person treating her, and I went along for a consultation. I was initially prescribed sepia pillules which had no effect whatsoever. Quite disappointed, after three weeks I informed Debbie that I still had industrial hot flushes, and was it worth continuing. She assured me it was, and then prescribed Sulphur pillules to take two three times a day. I looked Sulphur up on the Internet, and was quite impressed that it was prescribed to treat burning skin and throat 'catches' (amongst many others) which was exactly what I was suffering from. I looked forward to the miracle occurring of not suffering with either ailment any more. However, after some time it was evident that no miracle was going to happen as I still suffered on and off with the flushes and catches. I resigned myself to living with it, but the catches did lessen over time.

November 22nd was time for the usual annual MRI scan. I remembered only too well the year before how my head had to be encased in a vice just prior to my whole body going into the tunnel, and how noisy it all was. I looked to a repeat performance with dread. Phil, standing to one side of the scanner, could just about reach my hand in the tunnel and squeezed my fingers corresponding to how many more minutes I had left to endure in there. He had devised this routine as last year he remembered how I had told him I could not hear his voice in there due to the noise levels. Somehow with Phil's help I managed to stay in there without losing it.

I'm glad I managed to stay the distance. The oncologist was all smiles on December 6th when I attended the Nuffield hospital at Cambridge for the results. Thankfully I was still in remission. I would not need another appointment with her until December 2011. My usual appointment with the ENT surgeon for a check-up was scheduled for May, and the oncologist mentioned that there was a new ultrasound method of scanning that she would probably put me forward for when the next scan was due. I felt rather relieved that hopefully I wouldn't have to endure another MRI in 2011. My Christmas wasn't due to be spoiled this year! She also mentioned that she would refer me to a shoulder specialist if the tennis elbow operation did nothing to help the pain in my left arm and shoulder.

Christmas day was a time for celebrations with the family. Cousin Phillip and Uncle Harry came to visit Christmas morning, and Lee and Sarah came over with the girls on Christmas day afternoon and we opened presents. Late afternoon Phil, Mum and I went to Ipswich and were given a lovely Christmas dinner cooked by Anna's mother Alison. There were 12 of us all sitting round the table, and I felt so happy to be surrounded by such a lovely extended family. There were more presents to be opened after dinner, and poor Mum was happy but rather exhausted at the end of the day and virtually nodding off on her chair (well, she is 86!).

New Year's Eve was spent in London. Phil and I checked into the Strand Palace hotel during the afternoon, and after dinner walked down to the Embankment in order to secure a good spot to view the fireworks at midnight (everyone had had to get there early before the police put barriers up to stop too many people all trying to get to the same place). We had about a three-hour wait, but it was well worth it. We bagged a front row spot by the barrier, and the atmosphere was wonderful. When midnight struck the fireworks erupted from the London Eye and carried on for a good 10 minutes. It was only a short walk back to the hotel afterwards (instead of the usual two hour drive home) but it took ages due to the sheer number of people all trying to walk in the same direction.

By January 13th 2011 when the postponed operation on my left elbow was due, the pain in my left arm and shoulder had got much worse and the range of movement was reduced. I could not wait to get it over with to see if it would reduce the pain. I arrived on time at the BMI at Bury St. Edmunds. I was third on the list.

CHAPTER 35 - TENNIS ELBOW RELEASE

As I was not having a general anaesthetic (I had specifically requested a local) I had eaten some breakfast and was still sipping water when I arrived at the BMI. The admitting nurse looked rather worried until I reminded her that I was not going to be sedated.

The surgeon came to see me in my room beforehand, and I mentioned the trouble I was having trying to move my arm properly. There and then he diagnosed a frozen shoulder, and said that generally this problem goes away on its own over a period of time (usually about 2 years). He could inject the shoulder with steroid and local anaesthetic in clinic to help with pain relief, so I decided I would have the injection when I saw him for a post-op follow up appointment. Yet another complaint to cope with, and the annoying thing about this one was that I had not injured the shoulder at all and had no idea how I had done it (with hindsight I often wonder now if it was something to do with the major neck dissection operation).

In the anaesthetic room I was given 5 local injections around the elbow (a huge theatre assistant held my hand – how kind), and then was wheeled into the operating theatre and moved onto the high table (it was the first time in all my operations I had actually been awake at this point!). The operating theatre looked very frightening to somebody laid on the table at its mercy. The big overhead lights were switched on, and theatre assistants made sure that most of my body disappeared under a huge sterile cover (except my left arm). A screen was erected in front of me so that I could not see what was going on at the sharp end, and a tourniquet was put at the top of my arm before the surgeon made an incision. I felt no pain as the knife cut, but when he said he was 'scraping the bone to get rid of all the grey jelly that shouldn't be there' I started to feel quite a bit of pain (luckily this did not last too long). After about 20 minutes the procedure was over, my arm was bandaged up so that I could not straighten it, and then the tourniquet was removed. There was industrial pain and tingling for about half an hour after the tourniquet came off as the blood flowed back into my arm, and I spent this time in Recovery before being wheeled back to my room, where Phil remarked how much better I looked than before when I had been given a general anaesthetic.

I was allowed home after lunch, and would have to get used to doing everything one-handed for the following two weeks until the bandages came off. I had been given a foam support for my arm which I wore all day and took off at night, which helped as the arm could not be straightened and so could not hang down properly. I took Ibuprofen for a few days, as there was quite a bit of pain when the local anaesthetic wore off, and I had difficulty sleeping as I could not get comfortable. The left arm and hand were both warmer than the right, and the skin on my left hand was darker than the other one (I was told this was due to increased blood flow and was part of the healing process). As time wore on I had a terrible craving to straighten my arm out – the skin inside the elbow at the fold itched terribly, and I had to put a finger down inside the bandages to scratch the area and try to get some relief.

At last the two weeks passed and it was time to visit the surgeon for my post-op appointment. When the bandages and steri-strips came off, my arm looked withered and I could not straighten it at all. I panicked until the surgeon said this was quite normal, and that I should try and gently straighten it over time by letting it hang down as much as possible to lengthen the muscle again. The wound looked good and there was no infection. He would not do the shoulder injection at that point, as he said I had enough to be getting on with and to come back the following week for the injection. I would have liked to get it over with all at once, but was in quite a bit of pain so it probably made sense to wait before another assault on my body.

Over the next week my arm gradually straightened out, but was still thinner than the right arm, and for the first few days the skin was dry and kept flaking off. I rubbed grapeseed oil into the arm and over the wound, and by the time I went back for the shoulder injection the following week the arm did not look too bad, although it was still rather painful.

No wonder the surgeon had not wanted to do the shoulder injection at the same time; I have never known pain like it. The needle and syringe were huge, and afterwards I could barely lift my arm at all. I panicked again and wondered how I was going to drive home (Phil was away on business). I sat outside the hospital for about 45 minutes trying to move my arm enough to be able to change gear. I managed at long last to drive home, but was in terrible pain for a couple of days afterwards. However, after 2 days the pain started to subside and the shoulder was a little more flexible, as I suppose the steroid was helping with the inflammation. After about a week I could move the shoulder a lot more and the pain had greatly reduced, but I certainly did not fancy any more shoulder injections! I took six weeks off work by which time the elbow had healed and only a small scar was left, and the shoulder pain was a lot more bearable.

Soon after the shoulder injection I took the advice of the doctors in the Pain Clinic at work who always advocate core strengthening and Pilates for the overall general health of the muscles (particularly the back muscles). After a few months of doing these exercises I noticed an improvement in the low back pain I sometimes suffered from, and there was more movement in my left shoulder. After a day's typing at work I would often have pain in my left arm and shoulder, but 30 minutes of Pilates a day seemed to ease the problem. Overall the left shoulder remained slightly frozen though, but certainly a lot better than before the injection. Phil often massaged the shoulder and arm in the evenings, which also helped. Later in the year Phil bought a cross trainer, and this helped even more to strengthen my feeble arm muscles.

CHAPTER 36 – EVENTS IN 2011

Matt had been asked to go on tour for the whole of March as a guest guitarist with the band Aeon Zen who were supporting the Canadian musician Devin Townsend. He lived on a tour bus with 16 other musicians for a month and visited many different countries, playing to large venues and enthusiastic crowds. Gone were the days of playing to only a few people! He suffered the disrupted body clock, lack of sleep and hauling gear in and out of the venues in the early hours of the morning for the thrill of living the dream. He emerged thinner and wiser, and decided he'd only do it again if Anna could accompany him, and if there were more roadies employed to help with moving all the gear. We attended a couple of the gigs and had never seen him play to so many people.

Also in March Phil decided to change jobs after 21 years in the same one. With other things that had happened previously I wondered if possibly he was going through a male menopause in sympathy with mine, but he said he could not get on with the boss's son who had recently taken over the business and felt he could not continue there. He started working from home as European technical support for an American software company. What had been Matthew's bedroom before he left home became an office, and Phil seemed to thrive in his new workplace. There was not so much travelling in the new job either, as he gave technical advice by phone or by email, so that was an advantage too. The only disadvantage was that our medical insurance was now on an individual basis rather than a corporate one, so we had to contribute to some of the bills, but Phil's new company paid the monthly premiums.

My check up with the ENT surgeon was in May 2011 and once again all was well and no lumps were felt in my neck. Unfortunately he did not seem to know anything about the new ultrasound method of scanning, and thought it best that I have an MRI scan at the end of the year in the same machine that I had been in before for continuity. Also in May was a routine mammogram (my second – the first one was when I was 50) and also the first period I had had all year (thank goodness they were starting to fade away). The mammogram was normal, and the hot flushes started again in earnest after another period in July. The menopause was really beginning to bite.

Lee and Sarah started having problems with their neighbours in May, and unfortunately after having a brick thrown through their window and paint daubed on their car decided to put their house on the market. They were not allowed to increase their mortgage, so had to find somewhere to rent as they could not afford to move out of the area they were already in. My heart bled for them. If only I could win the lottery! Eventually it wasn't until October that they were able to move into a lovely rented three bedroomed house about three miles away from us. The girls were changed over to a local school, and they started to put all their troubles behind them. Fate wasn't that kind though, as soon after they moved in our eldest granddaughter Sophie started to have medical problems.

June and July was the festival season, and we did them proud: Download, Sonisphere, High Voltage, Hard Rock Calling in Hyde Park (where Bon Jovi played), and finally the Bestival festival on the Isle of Wight in September. I still had Jon Bon Jovi's email address from the previous year, and I sent him an email to say how much we had enjoyed the concert. His brother replied to say that Helen had reminded him that she and myself were still interested in helping set up the fan club. This was news to me as I thought it had all fallen through. Consequently we met up with Helen again at High Voltage, where she assured me that the Bon Jovi fan club job was still on and I would be hearing something after December. Jon Bon Jovi himself then sent me another email to say that there had been I.T problems and legal issues to resolve in the setting up of the fan club, but now he was setting up his own company to deal with it. Things were definitely looking up.

The Bestival saw us renewing our marriage vows in an inflatable church (but with a real vicar!) and with a congregation of Bestivallers looking on and cheering. We did not know any of them, but it did not seem to matter. I wore a long dress found for me in the dressing up tent next door, but we all kept our wellies on as it was a bit muddy! The wedding breakfast was in the Underground Restaurant opposite the church. Thankfully Bestival has so many surprises up its sleeve – the music is incidental as there are so many other things to do there (which is just as well as the music wasn't really to our taste). We love the Isle of Wight, want to retire there, and always seem to find something new to do every time we go there. We returned the following month for my birthday treat, and found a lovely clifftop walk at Compton Bay near Freshwater. You can look down at the beach below from the cliffs, and walk all the way into Freshwater if you've a mind to. We often look to the future and have decided that the best thing to do in retirement would be to sell our house and buy two flats with it, one here in East Anglia to be near the family, and one in the Isle of Wight. Then we would get the best of both worlds, but as retirement is at least another 10 years off, we would have to see how that pans out.

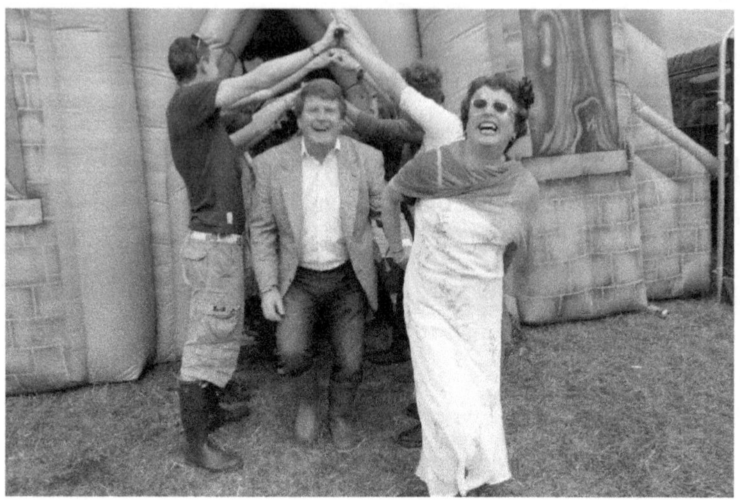

Phil and I getting married again at the Bestival – September 9th 2011.

We had a lovely holiday in Sorrento in October 2011, staying at the Hotel Capo di Monte just outside the town. The weather was just right (not too hot) and the scenery was superb. The Amalfi coast is just so beautiful, and we definitely want to return there at some point. The highlight for me was visiting Pompeii and Herculaneum and seeing for myself the damage incurred when Mount Vesuvius erupted in AD79. We walked up Mount Vesuvius, but I found my calf muscles hurt so much when I tried to walk down again (perhaps I'm just getting old or perhaps it was a rather steep descent!).

A friend at work had told me that wearing a 'Ladycare' magnet next to her skin had helped cure her of her menopausal hot flushes. I was interested enough to buy one, and found you had to wear it continually for at least three months for it to have any effect. Apparently it resolved the body's 'imbalance', and I prayed it would resolve mine. After three months I was still getting hot flushes unfortunately, but they had lessened in frequency so perhaps it did help a little bit. I continued wearing it.

I was rather worried about a small growth on the right side of my nose that I thought had been there for about six months or so. My GP was not sure if it was a rodent ulcer or not (this is a kind of skin cancer called a basal cell carcinoma that I was informed doesn't spread), so he decided to refer me to a dermatologist. The appointment came through for early December.

Some lovely news in November from Matt and Anna; their first child was due in May 2012. An early scan showed things were progressing normally, although they could not see the sex of the child. We would soon be grandparents three times over!

Our first grandchild Sophie was now aged 6, and suddenly she was waking night after night with a racing heart, sweats and shakes. We were all understandably very worried. The GP could hear a heart murmur, and referred her to the paediatric cardiologist who diagnosed supraventricular tachycardia (SVT) after she had worn a 24 hour monitor. The only way to rectify this condition was by surgery. Poor little Sophie, so young to have to possibly undergo a heart operation.

My yearly MRI scan was due on November 30th, with a visit to the oncologist a few days after for the results. Once again I had to shut my eyes in the scanner, especially when I felt the cage going over my face to start with. It really is the most unpleasant experience. Phil was there to hold my hand again, and it was reassuring to know he was there (I have a fear of being stuck in there!).

A few days after the scan was my annual check-up with the oncologist. This was the penultimate time I would see her privately, as the insurance company would only pay for five years of follow ups, and this would cease in October 2012. Happily I was still in remission. I asked her to have a look at the possible rodent ulcer on the side of my nose. She was not sure what it was either, but reassured me if it was a rodent ulcer it would not spread, and the GP was doing the right thing in referring me to a dermatologist where it could be taken off with a local anaesthetic. We made another appointment for 8th October 2012.

The dermatologist was certain that I had a rodent ulcer, and she referred me to a plastic surgeon to have it removed. Apparently this type of skin cancer is caused by sun damage and is very common, but she reassured me that it does not spread around the body like a malignant melanoma would. A rodent ulcer gnaws away at the surrounding tissue and just gets bigger and bigger. It was time though for it to come off. I was 'lucky' in that I had had two different types of cancer that were treatable. I wondered if I would be so lucky if it happened again a third time.

Lee kindly took me to the BMI at Bury St Edmunds on the morning of the procedure a couple of days before Christmas. Phil had not been in his new job that long, and it was not as easy as before to take time off at short notice.

The plastic surgeon came to have a look at me. He marked out the place with a marker that required removing, and explained to me that he would have to take a slightly larger area away to ensure the whole cancer was removed (it would be sent off for biopsy to confirm all the margins were intact). As he was speaking there was a big heartsink moment as I realised I would have quite a bigger scar on my face than I had anticipated (it was a 'necessary evil' according to the surgeon). He then asked me to sign the consent forms, administered the local anaesthetic, and I then walked into the theatre with the nurse for the procedure.

It's really quite scary lying wide awake on the operating table (for the second time this year!). I felt just like a slab of meat in the butcher's shop. The lights above me were so bright that it was like looking into the sun. The nurse placed some gauze over my eyes to stop me squinting, and the surgeon went to work. There was some soothing classical music in the background, and apart from the surgeon's quiet statements to the nurse requesting various instruments, there was not much other noise. After about half an hour he told me that he had placed 18 stitches on the outside of the skin (there were some dissolvable internal stitches) and some sterile dressings, and that he had finished and I could walk back to my room. I felt a bit shaky when I went to stand up, and was glad to reach my room to have a bit of a rest before asking Phil to come and collect me.

Unfortunately all of Christmas was spent with a big black eye, as the bruising started to come out. Apart from that the Christmas break was very good; I cooked dinner on Christmas Day for Lee, Sarah and girls, Matt and Anna and my Mum, and it was great to have everybody together. On Boxing Day we had my cousin Phillip come to visit us and Matt and Anna, and we visited Anna's parents on the evenings of Christmas Day and Boxing Day.

On 28th December I visited the GP surgery to have the stitches taken out by a practice nurse. She remarked that part of the scar was still a bit 'gappy' and after taking out the stitches she put some steri-strips over the gappy part. After another week had passed the majority of the scar was healing nicely, but the part of the scar where the steri-strips had been applied (directly under my eye) had still not closed properly, although it had healed. I contacted the surgeon's secretary and she made me an appointment to come back and see him on 9th January so that he could have a look at it and make a decision as to what to do about it.

New Year's Eve was spent on a riverboat cruise up the Thames to see the fireworks at midnight. There was a wonderful atmosphere created by a quarter of a million people, and the fireworks were amazing. There was a downside to it though, as we were late getting off the boat and it took over an hour to walk the short distance back to our hotel in the Strand as the police had barricaded many roads off, making them impassable (the previous year we managed to return to the hotel a lot sooner as we had left as soon as the fireworks finished). This caused a build-up of people at the few roads that were passable, making a bit of a crush. Nevertheless we arrived with some relief at the Strand Palace hotel at about 1.30am on New Year's Day.

CHAPTER 37 – EVENTS IN 2012

On 9th January 2012 I re-presented to the surgeon. He said there were some remnants of sutures in the top part of the scar, which was why it was not closing properly. He cleaned it out and said it would heal with time but might leave a 'groove' (apparently it did not need any more stitches or steri-strips). He could repair the groove if I wanted to go through another procedure with local anaesthetic again. I decided to try massaging the scar with bio-oil for three months to see if that helped the healing process. It seemed to, and after three months or so the scarring was certainly less visible. I decided not to go back to the surgeon for the follow up appointment and was thankful my face did not look too much like a map of the Norfolk broads.

Unfortunately in February my right eye started to become sore (oh no, not again). It did not feel like the left eye did three years previously though, as it was not watering and I did not have conjunctivitis-like symptoms. However, the only thing that stopped the soreness were the chloramphenicol eye drops that were still on repeat prescription from three years ago. When I had another attack in March on a weekend away in London, I decided to visit the same ophthalmologist that had diagnosed the symptoms in the left eye (the left eye was still ok and the DCR was still working well) and had found the link between radioiodine and narrowing of the naso-lachrymal duct. I had a feeling it was not quite the same problem though as the eye was not constantly watering and I could taste the chloramphenicol at the back of my throat after applying it to the right eye, so the naso-lachrymal duct on the right side was apparently working as it should. The right eye felt very dry sometimes though, especially in the mornings, and sometimes my vision in that eye was cloudy.

The ophthalmologist seemed to remember me from 2009 (I was probably becoming notorious in medical circles). He had a look at the inside of the eye and syringed the tear duct, which seemed to be working as it should. He diagnosed blepharitis and said the glands in the lids of the eyes sometimes overproduce oil which collects on the cornea and needs to be broken up. He prescribed some sterile drops called Celluvisc which would do the job of breaking up the oil and making my vision less cloudy in the mornings (I could use up to 8 drops a day as and when required). He also prescribed some Blephaclean wipes which I needed to apply to the lids once a day. Surprisingly it worked. The GP added them onto my repeat prescriptions, and I was relieved that I did not need another DCR. I started to use the Celluvisc during the night if I woke up, and it seemed to do the trick.

There had been no news regarding the Jon Bon Jovi fan club. I hoped and hoped that I would get an email, but nothing arrived. Helen thought that maybe nothing was going to happen after all.

On a happier note, Sophie was gaining weight and was not having so many SVT attacks. The cardiologist decided not to operate, but to monitor her and for her to come back and see him if the attacks started again. Matthew had been born with a heart murmur but grew out of it, so perhaps the same would happen for Sophie.

My mother's 88th birthday was due on May 21st. The previous day the family all gathered together for a pub lunch to celebrate. Anna was hugely pregnant, and when I looked at her I knew somehow that the baby would be born the next day. Sure enough little William was born at 5.50am on Mum's birthday – all 7lb 9 and a half ounces of him. He was gorgeous and looked just like his daddy.

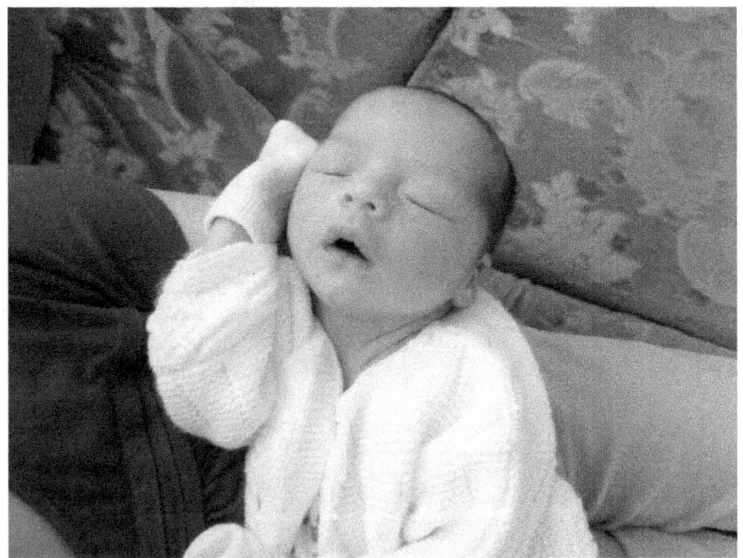

William Shepherd aged two days

The summer of 2012 was dismal as far as the weather was concerned. The Download festival and Isle of Wight festival were absolute mudbaths, especially Download. I have a vivid memory of trying to lift my boots in the thick mud to try and walk, but it was proving very difficult. Luckily my eldest son Lee and his friend were on hand to help, as you can see below!

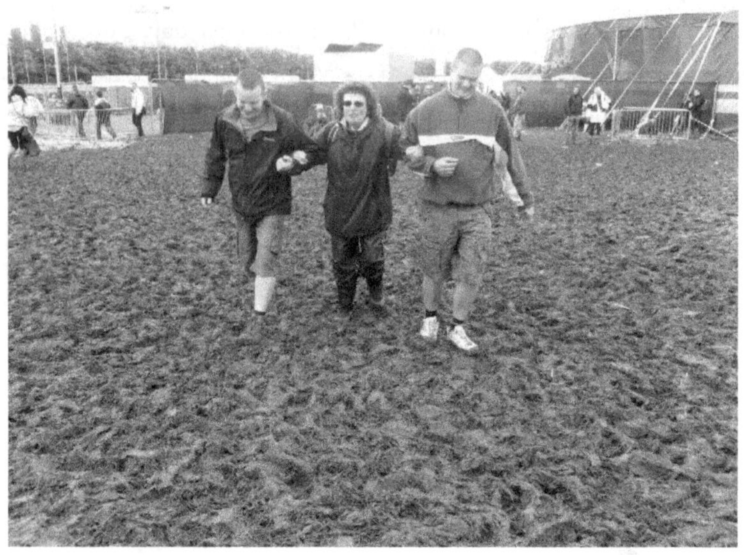

On July 1ˢᵗ myself, Phil, Matt, Anna (and William) and some friends from work did a 4 mile charity walk in aid of the British Thyroid Foundation. This was the second walk that I had organised – the first being a year previously. The weather was surprisingly good that day, and we made £267 in sponsorship money (my cousin Phillip had very generously given £100!). This figure however was about £100 down on the year before, but I enjoyed organising it and was pleased to help the BTF.

On July 27ᵗʰ Lee turned 30. Sarah and I had organised a surprise party for him that was held in a pub in their village. Over 50 people attended – family and friends, and there was a bungee run in the pub garden. Everybody had managed to keep it a secret from Lee, and it was lovely to see the look of surprise on his face. Anna had very cleverly arranged William's christening for the following day, when all the family were staying nearby overnight. William was as good as gold all through the service, and there was a buffet afterwards at the school where Anna teaches, organised by Anna herself with some help from her mum.

On September 1st Phil and I flew out to Majorca to holiday at the Playa Hotel at Camp de Mar. It was a peaceful and quiet resort, and we had a lovely holiday. We visited the Caves of Drach (where we had taken the boys 15 years before when staying at Alcudia), the Basilica at Lluc, and took a tram ride at Soller that took us to Palma. We swam in the clear warm sea at Camp de Mar, and saved bread from the hotel's dining room to feed the fishes that we saw swimming around us. It was idyllic.

Soon after returning it was time for the yearly MRI scan. It had been brought forward this year to September because my insurance company had declared that my insurance policy would terminate at the end of September. They had paid for four years of follow ups for me, and this year would be the fifth and last. However, if I needed treatment they would happily pay for it, but not for any more follow ups.

Phil came with me for the hated MRI scan, and held my hand in the scanner. We had devised a code whereby if he squeezed my hand five times I knew the scan would last another five minutes, four squeezes for four minutes, and so on. It was so noisy in there that I could not hear anything he said, so the squeezing worked well for us. Once again I had to keep my eyes shut to endure it (I felt something being put over my head and neck, but dared not look otherwise I felt I would panic if I opened my eyes and found I was enclosed).

My appointment with the oncologist was at the end of September before the policy ran out. Happily I was still in remission, and I breathed a sigh of relief as I walked out of the door. My latest blood test showed that I was a little over-replaced on thyroxine, and had to reduce it a bit to 125mcg three times a week and 150mcg for the other four days. I'd also had a blood test to check on the level of thyroglobulin antibodies, which fortunately were still on the downward trend at 231 (two years' previously this result had been

342). This was further proof that the cancer was still in remission. My next appointment would be on the NHS on 1st October 2013 at Addenbrooke's Thyroid Clinic.

Unfortunately this good news was tinged with sadness, as without going into too much detail, in the last half of 2012 I started to go through a very troublesome time, which caused me much stress (it was nothing to do with cancer). The problem had been looming for some years, and as the year progressed I found that I could not concentrate at work at all, and as the problem came to a head it seemed all-consuming at the time and I could think of nothing else. I must have started to make mistakes, because the happy 7-year working relationship between myself and the doctor I worked for suddenly started to break down. I felt I could not approach anybody at work with my problem, and when the opportunity came to take up a post in a different department I jumped at the chance. The new post would not become available until later in 2013, and so I decided to take a few months off work to write about my problem and pour out my heart into a work of fiction as a form of therapy. With the exception of the doctor I worked for, all of my work colleagues were very upset that I was leaving. It was a very sad time for me.

At Christmas time there was a lovely dinner at Anna's parents' house on Christmas Day, and then all the family came to us for tea on Boxing Day. On New Years' Eve Phil and I bought tickets for a dinner, dance and fireworks at a local hotel. I did not feel like celebrating in London this time, and wanted something a little quieter instead.

CHAPTER 38 - EVENTS IN 2013

I started to write my fiction book soon after Christmas while I was off work (I used a pen name). I looked on the bright side; I had been given the chance to do something I loved. Writing was a wonderful therapy, and when the book was finished in February 2013 I sent off the first few chapters to a couple of prospective literary agents. By March 2013 I had heard back from one New York agent who said it was the best new story she had read in a long time, but that I needed to re-write it in the third person and in the present tense so that it was less like a memoir and more like a story (I had used the past tense and the first person). I eventually rewrote it and self-published it under a pseudonym, and to this day it is selling quite a few copies. The agent was right; the new version was considerably better than the original, but as any new author will tell you, finding a literary agent is akin to finding a pot of gold at the end of a rainbow.

The encouragement I received from various literary agents started me out on the road to writing fiction in my spare time. I kept the pen name I used with my first book, and to date have written five novels. They are all self-published and sell a few copies each month. I am never going to be up there with the big authors, but I have found a hobby that I love and who knows, one day I may even acquire a literary agent and be able to write full time!

In February 2013, Phil and I went out for a Valentine's Day dinner to Café Rouge and decided to have lobster soup for starters.

He had never eaten lobster before and had a really bad reaction right there in front of me in the restaurant, fainting and vomiting within half an hour of eating the soup. I'd never seen anything like it and at one point thought he'd died in the chair (he's never fainted before, and is usually hale and hearty). A visit to A&E could find nothing wrong except his usual slow heartbeat. An echocardiogram was requested, which showed an abnormal valve in his heart, which was probably congenital but had never caused him any problems and he was told it had not contributed to his fainting episode. Allergy tests at Addenbrooke's were inconclusive. We were no further forward.

We had decided our 2013 holiday would be visiting Toronto with Matt and Anna. Some of Anna's relatives live there, and we booked the flights in February. We would be flying out from Gatwick airport on August 10th. I looked forward to seeing Niagara Falls.

In the meantime granddaughter Sophie had to wear a heart monitor for a week in May. This had been requested some weeks' previously when she had suffered from some more palpitations. She was investigated for Woolf-Parkinson-White syndrome, but results were inconclusive. I too often had palpitations when I ate certain foods, and wondered if she had a food allergy. Fortunately for Sophie, she was given the all–clear eventually, and carried on running around full of her usual energy.

I had also began to suffer with quite frequent low back pain, and my GP requested an MRI scan. I stated my preference for this to be done at Addenbrooke's hospital, as I did not want to have treatment in the Pain Department where I had worked from the doctor that was not talking to me! I was doing my best to strengthen my core muscles by attending Pilates classes, but the back pain was still niggling and sometimes the muscles at the bottom of my back would go into painful spasm if I forgot to bend at the knees and keep my back straight when picking something up from the floor. I assumed the pain was down to arthritis of the spine / ageing, but the GP wanted to make sure the cancer hadn't spread to the bones. My oncologist assured her that no recurrence had been seen on the last MRI scan. A bone density scan was also requested.

I duly attended for the bone density scan (performed locally in the Nuffield hospital in Bury St. Edmunds) and for my first appointment in the Back Pain Clinic at Addenbrooke's in June 2013 just before our visit to the Isle of Wight festival. To my horror, the bone density report came back with a 10% bone loss at the base of the spine. I had been warned of the possible occurrence of osteoporosis by my oncologist soon after she had started me on the high dose thyroxine regime, but this was proof on paper that I had the forerunner of brittle bone disease. Apparently I was 'osteopenic', and I would need a 5 year treatment plan with bisphosphonates to harden my bones.

I looked up 'bisphosphonates' on Google. Horrified I saw that the tablets could cause necrosis of the jaw, cancer of the oesophagus, and augment any reflux or GI problems. The tablets could only be taken on an empty stomach in the morning, and one had to stay upright for at least an hour after a tablet had been taken. There were yearly injections if the tablets could not be tolerated. Straight away I phoned my insurance company to find out if I could have injections privately. I suffered with reflux, and obviously already had a predisposition to cancer. They requested a medical report from my GP. The weeks dragged by while the report was typed and sent to my insurance company. Eventually I was given an appointment to see a rheumatologist privately.

The rheumatologist explained again that I had the forerunner of osteoporosis, which was probably caused by the high doses of thyroxine I had taken in the past to keep the TSH suppressed. He asked my GP to refer me to him on the NHS, as the infusion was not done in private hospitals. He explained that I should get my teeth checked out at the dentist beforehand, as there was a rare chance that any tooth removal or root canal work could lead to necrosis of the jaw, and that the infusion could make me feel 'achey and fluey' for a couple of days afterwards.

At the Addenbrooke's Back Pain Clinic I was seen and examined by a spinal physiotherapist who thought I had some wear and tear due to age at the bottom of my spine, but that an MRI scan was not required. She asked the GP to perform some blood tests to check for inflammation, and also to check for low vitamin D levels. The vitamin D level came back low, and I was placed on a week's very high dose of vitamin D, and thereafter given Adcal D3 tablets to chew twice a day. These were a combined therapy for the bones of calcium and vitamin D.

I was a few days into the high dose vitamin D regime when I began to experience tinnitus and frequent heart palpitations, the palpitations occurring about twice every minute. They did not go away and were still there when I boarded the plane to Toronto with Phil, Matt, Anna and William on August 10th. I did not feel dizzy or anything dramatic, but the wonderful holiday we had helped me to put them to the back of my mind.

We visited Kincardine, laid on the sand at Bruce Beach, and then visited Anna's relatives in Toronto and Ottawa. We then went back in time and stayed at a 100 year old farmhouse up near Algonquin Park, and introduced William to the horses, hens and various kittens and dogs there. The weather stayed fine and we cooked our own food on the farmhouse BBQ every night and ate al fresco, with the kittens hoovering up the leftovers. Then it was time to head down to Niagara and see the falls, the Skylon Tower, and all that Clifton Hill had to offer.

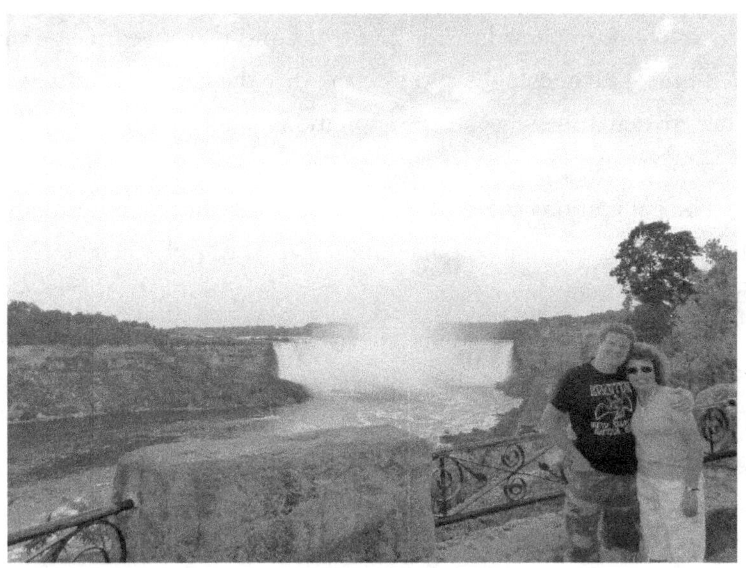

Phil and I at Niagara Falls August 2013

When we came home I still had the heart palpitations, and I sometimes felt shaky. I had another blood test and I was still too over-replaced on thyroxine, so I had to cut it down yet again to 100mcg daily. I wondered if it was the high dose of thyroxine or the high dose of vitamin D that was causing the palpitations. I had an ECG and was told I had ectopic beats that were not dangerous in any way.

It was also time to go back to work to start in a new department, and I was dreading it. The job I was originally told was mine was no longer available, and I was put into the dermatology department. The workload was phenomenal, and my elbows started to suffer again with the increased amount of typing I had to do. However, the people were lovely which made things a little easier.

My check up with the oncologist at Addenbrooke's came around at the beginning of October. This time I joined the 70 or so other patients who were due to see her that day on the NHS. She felt my neck and assured me she could not feel any lumps. I had more blood tests to check my new level of thyroxine, and these eventually came back fine. The oncologist also told me that she had heard of several other patients having heart palpitations after taking high-dose vitamin D.

The palpitations eventually settled down about two months after the high-dose vitamin D course, and I started to feel much better on the lower dose of thyroxine.

At the end of October I had an appointment for my bisphosphonate infusion. Feeling nervous I turned up at the Medical Treatment Unit of the hospital where I work, but was pleasantly relieved to feel no symptoms from the infusion or for the few hours afterwards. The procedure only took about 20 minutes, and as soon as I was disconnected from the drip I was allowed home.

However, things changed suddenly when I woke up at 1am the next morning. I had never felt my heart beating so fast before; something was not right. I got out of bed and felt weak and was trembling. My face was blood red. Phil was away and I was alone. I phoned 999 and asked for an ambulance; I felt dreadful. They asked me to take my pulse; it was 160 beats per minute.

The ambulance took half an hour to arrive. The paramedics did an ECG and told me I had sinus tachycardia. My heart rate was too rapid for me to remain at home, and so they took me to A&E at the hospital where I work. The A&E doctor assured me all bloods taken were fine; I just had to ride it out and wait for the reaction to wear off. I paid for a taxi home and slept for most of the following day.

The following night I was up again twice in the night inhaling Vick fumes, with thick phlegm stuck at the back of my throat. My heart rate had subsided a bit, to about 100 beats per minute, but I still did not feel well. To think I had to undergo another four of these infusions!

My heart rate eventually settled down, but the palpitations came back with a vengeance. I experimented, and found that every time I stopped taking the Adcal D3 tablets the palpitations went away after about a week, but returned soon after taking the tablets again. I finally decided to stop taking them and bought a calcium supplement which did not have vitamin D added from the health food shop instead, which my body tolerated better. I also went to the GP and was checked with an echocardiogram and a 24 hour tape. The good news came back that my heart was structurally sound, and all that was found were a few ectopic beats.

CHAPTER 39 - 2014

So here we are in 2014. As of June this year I am still in remission, but continue to have yearly check-ups and an MRI scan every 2 years. The thick phlegm at the back of my throat only appears if I have bisphosphonate infusions or if I catch a cold, and the frequent eye infections are thankfully now in the past due to having had a DCR operation. However, I still have dry eyes at night, and manage this condition by using Celluvisc eye drops.

Hopefully the thyroxine tablets I have no choice but to take will not cause osteoporosis, as I am now having the yearly bisphosphonate infusions and taking calcium supplements. My body seems to be okay now on 100mcg of thyroxine, and I am only hot some of the time instead of all of the time. I am almost through the menopause and out the other side, and only get a few hot flushes per day now. What a relief it is to be free of PMT and periods! I enjoy my work, and when I am not typing clinic letters I am writing fiction.

I try and help my tendency for low back pain by doing daily Pilates exercises,

by attending a Pilates class once a week, and by walking for at least half an hour each day and keeping my weight down. I can no longer jog, as my left knee would let me know about it if I did, but I have learned through working in the Pain Department that to be happy in this life you have to learn to accept the 'new normal'. I have typed so many clinic letters of patients unhappy that they cannot do in middle-age what they used to do when they were young, that it sunk into my brain to accept the limitations of an ageing body and make the best of what you have.

The film company 'Coast' will be filming me on 31st May, as they think I am a good candidate to give hope to other thyroid cancer sufferers. Phil and I will be celebrating our 34th wedding anniversary this year, and also attending the Isle of Wight Festival and the Sonisphere Festival. When my legs ache I will sit on the grass, listen to the bands, and thank the good Lord up above that I am still alive!

BOOK 3

2014 ONWARDS

CHAPTER 40 – RETURN OF THYROID CANCER

I suppose I had become rather blasé about the whole thyroid cancer thing. Whilst waiting to see the oncologist in her NHS clinic in early October 2014, I sat patiently reading my Kindle and waiting for my name to be called. All my previous check-up appointments since December 2007 had been fine, and almost seven years down the line I had no doubts at all that this latest follow up would be exactly the same.

The clinic was running over an hour late. There were 70 patients on the list to be seen, and I was one of them. After five years of follow ups, my insurance company had informed me that they would not be paying for any more check-ups, and so it was to the large NHS thyroid clinic at Addenbrooke's Hospital that I had driven that morning, which was about 50 miles from my home in Suffolk.

As I sat there wondering when it would be my turn, I looked around at some of the other patients and felt relief that I had finally shaken the disease free some time ago. I saw the lines of worry on the faces, and did not envy them the surgery, radiation, and possibly more surgery that they would have to endure to get to the stage where I was now at.

At last the nurse called my name and ushered me to another waiting area just outside the consultant's office. I smiled at her as I sat down and picked up my Kindle again. However, the wait was brief this time, and about an hour and a half after my appointment time I was finally called in.

Usually the oncologist would inform me that my latest MRI was fine almost before I had sat down. This time I noticed a nurse was present. The oncologist did not mention the results of the MRI at all, and instead asked me about how much thyroxine I was taking, and whether I had good energy levels. A little warning bell started up in my brain, and I asked her for the results of the MRI scan. She replied that she would 'get to that in a minute'.

As soon as I heard those words I knew something was wrong. My heart sank and I quickly looked over at the thyroid cancer nurse, whose expression was inscrutable. I sighed, put on a brave face, and waited impatiently to hear my fate.

The oncologist tried to break me in gently, but when she informed me of two lymph nodes that had increased in size on the right side of my neck, I knew the cancer had returned. Thankfully the left side which had undergone a radical neck dissection in 2007 was still clear, but the unaffected right side was now of some concern.

I asked the consultant whether the myriad of insect bites I had suffered over the summer could have caused the lymph nodes to enlarge. She nodded and said this was possible, but she had discussed my case at a multi-disciplinary meeting that morning, and to be on the safe side she wanted me to have a detailed ultrasound scan and fine needle biopsy, and to come back and see her in a month's time for the results.

Silently I nodded in agreement, and could not wait to get out of the consultation room. My husband Phil was not with me, as for the past few years I had told him not to bother coming along to all my routine check-ups. He now mostly worked at home as technical support for an American company, but thankfully was not out travelling that day. My eyes filled with tears as I talked to him on my mobile phone whilst walking back to the car park. He agreed the ultrasound and biopsy were needed just to make sure that the enlarged nodes were not caused by insect bites. He told me to think positive.

This is not a very easy thing to do, and I then had a terrible three weeks waiting for the ultrasound appointment. It seems to be worse on the run-up to Christmas, when all the family are cheerfully looking forward to time off work and getting together for lunches and dinners. My daughters-in-law tried to sort out Christmas arrangements with me, but my mind was elsewhere and I kept forgetting what they were telling me. I could not think past October 28th, which was the date my ultrasound scan was booked for. Coincidentally it was also my birthday, and I was keeping fingers and toes crossed for a good result.

Unfortunately the good result was not to be. I had the worst birthday ever as the radiologist doing the scan gently informed me that he did not need to perform a biopsy, as he could see papillary thyroid cancer on the right side of my neck, and possibly some more down near the thyroid bed, but the latter could have been just due to scarring. He assured me the lymph nodes were only small and that the cancer had had been detected early, but also told me that they needed to be taken out.

I lay on the couch, closed my eyes, and tried not to cry in front of the radiologist, but on the way back to the car the tears started to flow. When I got home Phil gave me a cuddle and reiterated that the lymph nodes were only small and that there only seemed to be two of them, but that was two too many as far as I was concerned.

After the ultrasound came the bit about telling the family that I needed more surgery on my neck. At the time my mother was 90 years old and very frail, but fully compos mentis. My eldest son Lee lived nearby with his wife Sarah and their two daughters, and my youngest son Matthew lived with his wife Anna and their son William about 25 miles away. Anna was also pregnant with our fourth grandchild. I hated telling them, but had to do it.

Mum said that she would pray for me. Lee cuddled me and started my tears falling again, and Matthew asked lots of questions on the phone and gave me an extra cuddle when I saw him. I could hardly believe that I was messing up their Christmases all over again.

The next appointment with the oncologist was on 4th November. I wanted to ask her whether the cancer had returned due to me having to reduce my thyroxine dose to counterbalance the osteopenia (the very early stage of osteoporosis) and palpitations that I was now suffering from, caused by too much thyroxine. I also wanted to ask her if she thought there may be other cancerous lymph nodes elsewhere in my body apart from the small non-growing nodules in the lungs that we already knew about.

I waited with Phil for about 45 minutes in the thyroid clinic to see the oncologist on the day of my appointment. She asked me what I had learned from the radiologist, and reiterated his news that I needed to be seen by the ENT surgeon who had performed my left neck dissection in 2007. This time I would need a right neck dissection to remove 2 lymph nodes in the right side of the neck, and a small amount of suspicious-looking tissue in the thyroid bed. After my surgery I would need to see the oncologist again for a PET / CT scan, to make sure there were no other cancerous lymph nodes elsewhere in my body.

Deep joy.

I asked her whether I should increase my thyroxine dose, and she shook her head. Apparently it is important to make sure long-term thyroxine patients are not having their thyroid stimulating hormone too over-suppressed with large doses of thyroxine, as the extra thyroxine in the body causes low bone density and palpitations, something I had started to suffer from. I was due to have another bone scan in January 2015 to ensure that my lower back was not losing too much bone, but was feeling better regarding the palpitations with taking a lower dose of thyroxine.

Coincidentally my British Thyroid Foundation magazine was delivered around this time, and I read of the effect of calcium on the thyroid stimulating hormone level (TSH). My TSH had been slightly raised from previous levels, and it started me thinking whether my daily calcium tablets were affecting my TSH levels as well as the reduced thyroxine. Apparently oestrogen also raised TSH levels; I had been seriously considering starting HRT to help with my low bone density, and to read this was like having a slap in the face.

I was still feeling the after-effects of previous thyroid cancer treatment, and did not relish any more. The thought of more surgery made me feel terribly depressed, and I could not seem to concentrate on my usual pastime of writing women's fiction novels. I had just finished my seventh book (under my usual pen name), and decided to start writing this book instead as a form of therapy.

Leafing through my first book 'Thyroid Cancer for Beginners', I gave a wry smile at the few sentences I had written describing a fellow thyroid cancer sufferer's neck in the clinic as being like a 'map of the Norfolk Broads'. I had not long had my thyroidectomy at the time, and only had a small scar across the base of my neck. Little did I know what was waiting for me – my own neck would soon be just as scarred. Perhaps I should have kept my mouth shut……

CHAPTER 41 – RIGHT NECK DISSECTION

The surgeon greeted me with a smile as I walked into the consultation room on 10th November. I hadn't seen him for a couple of years as he had stopped working at my hospital and my insurance company had stopped paying for any further follow-ups, but he still remembered me.

He felt around my neck and was convinced that he could feel the two lymph nodes in question on the right side of my neck, although they were very small. He assured me that the cancer was slow-growing and there was no real urgency for the operation, but said if I did not have the surgery then the nodes would grow bigger. I agreed to him performing the operation on 4th December, and was secretly relieved that I didn't have to go to work over the Christmas period. He inserted the hated camera up my nose to ensure my right vocal cord was still working – it was.

The surgeon thought that the operation this time would not take as long as when he did the left side, as there was less work for him to do. He mentioned there was a 'big lump' previously that he had had to take out of the thyroid bed on the left side, and that had taken quite a few of the 6 hours that I was under the anaesthetic. He did say there was still a 'small area' in the thyroid bed that he would need to remove, but that it was a much smaller area than last time and he wasn't even sure it was cancerous tissue. It could be just scar tissue, but he would not be sure until after it was removed and biopsied.

This was the first time I had heard about any previous recurrence in the thyroid bed. I realised then that information is kept back by the doctors, and patients only hear what doctors want them to hear.

I asked about the altered sensation and slight pain I had been experiencing on the left side of my neck over the previous fortnight or so. Like the oncologist, the surgeon had no idea what was causing it. I put it down to ageing or maybe adhesions from the effects of the previous surgery.

The time dragged slowly towards Thursday December 4th. On the Tuesday before I attended the pre-assessment clinic at the Cambridge Nuffield hospital, about 50 miles away, where my blood pressure, height, weight and urine were checked, along with swabs for MRSA. I was pleased to incidentally find out that my BMI was normal at 24.

Apparently the anaesthetist had already checked in earlier that day, eager to find out about his nightmare job….me (the patient with the reduced airway and increased phlegm afterwards). The day before I filled up the fridge with food, wrote a bit more of my eighth novel, packed my bag ready for the journey, and received messages from well-wishers.

I was due in Theatre at 1.30pm. At eleven o'clock on the fateful day we left home to return to the Cambridge Nuffield. I had packed various things to keep me occupied, and when I was shown to room number 225, I tried to concentrate on my Kindle book whilst various nurses bustled about filling out admission forms and handing me the mandatory backside-showing hospital gown and anti-DVT stockings. My blood pressure was through the roof with nerves, and I was thirsty and shaky and cold through lack of food.

Then came more visitors; the surgeon came in to take my consent and explain about all the things that could go wrong. The anaesthetist popped his head around the door and I took the chance to explain my reduced airway through having only one working vocal cord, also the increased phlegm after a general anaesthetic, and of sleep apnoea if I am asleep/unconscious and am lying flat on my back. The anaesthetist did not seem bothered by all this, and said he would use a special tube to intubate me that went down my windpipe. He was present at the previous operation, and remembered me from 7 years before when the left side of my neck was dissected, and so had all my notes. I reminded him that when I had woken up after the previous operation I had never felt so hot in my life. He reassured me he would keep an eye on my body temperature.

As I donned my unflattering gown and paper knickers I sighed with the knowledge I had gained through undergoing the first neck dissection and thyroidectomy. I knew I would be awake for the next 3 days and nights, and would also need nebulisers for three days after the operation to try and shift the increased phlegm, and I remembered that it always took me at least 7 days to recover from a general anaesthetic (or liquid cosh as it can sometimes be known). I was not looking forward to the procedure at all, and could still hardly believe that I was having to go through it all again; this time would be the third major operation on my neck.

An emergency child's operation had been slotted in before mine, so it was not until 3pm that I was able to put on the dressing gown provided and walk to the operating theatre. Phil took my slippers and glasses at the door to the anaesthetic room and gave me a kiss, and by then my adrenaline was running so high that my fingertips were tingling. I lay down on the narrow trolley while a cannula was put in my hand by the anaesthetist who had visited my room earlier. As the cosh started flowing through my veins I felt something shut down in my brain, and for just a few seconds before lights out I knew why the addicts were so keen to get their hands on such powerful narcotics (you just don't care about anything anymore!).

It seemed as though no sooner had I gone to sleep than I was waking up in Recovery. However, six hours had passed, and the waking up process was to take several hours instead of a few moments. I realised I did not feel as hot as the previous time though, and silently thanked the anaesthetist for his diligence.

My brain was firing but I could not articulate, and a combination of all the drugs I had been given had caused a migraine on top of everything else. I reached up with my right hand to feel the wound, but somebody gently moved it down again. Then I was somehow back in my room, but I do not remember arriving. The clock showed ten minutes past nine in the evening. Phil held my hand and gave me a sip of water.

A blood pressure cuff was attached to my arm, which inflated and deflated at regular intervals. There was one chest drain in place. Nurses hurried in and out taking observations every 15 minutes, and I suddenly became aware that my bladder was feeling very full. I was still hooked up to a drip for hydration, and I most definitely needed a wee. As Phil did that terribly unromantic thing again and lifted me onto a bedpan, my head swum around and I wondered if I was going to be sick. I managed to blurt out that I was nauseous, and an anti-emetic was given through the cannula. Thankfully the nausea then began to reduce.

I vaguely remember seeing the anaesthetist come in to check how I was getting on, but the surgeon did not reappear. The anaesthetist informed me the operation had gone well, and that several nodes had been taken out and had been sent away for analysis. I thanked him for his work and felt somewhat guilty for keeping him at the hospital so late into the evening.

I continued sipping water and waking up. My neck felt stiff and sore, and I was weak and shaky. Phil stayed by my bedside for the entire long night, and once more became King of the Bedpans whilst I was still hooked up to the drip.

On the second day (Friday 5th December) the hydration drip was taken away, and I was grateful to be able to nibble on a piece of toast. I managed to hobble to the toilet, and had a little wash at the sink. When I looked at myself in the mirror I resembled death on legs, but marvelled at the neat job the surgeon had done with the multitude of metal clips keeping the wound together. My voice was worryingly weak, but when the surgeon visited he said it would settle down in time, and the weakness was probably either due to bruising and swelling, or having the endotracheal tube inserted during intubation.

I started on the prescribed nebulisers to counteract the build-up of phlegm and mucus caused by the anaesthetic gases. By Saturday I could walk around in the corridor outside, and eagerly awaited the surgeon's verdict as to when I could return home. Unfortunately the drain was still producing too many secretions, and I had to wait until the Sunday evening before it was finally taken out and I was able to leave.

Back at home it took a good week for the mucus to clear and for me to feel at least partly normal. At last I could sleep for short periods though, which is impossible in a hospital environment due to nurses, cleaners, doctors and the rest of the world waltzing in and out of my room every five minutes. I was forgetful, and at one point wondered if I had early Alzheimer's. I was also weak, tired, and in quite a bit of pain, and so kept up with the Ibuprofen and Paracetamol that had been started after the operation. Phil took a couple of days off work and was there to help me rehabilitate and mobilise again. By the sixth day I had started to walk outside around our village. It was wonderful to feel the sun on my face again.

CHAPTER 42 – RESULT OF BIOPSY AND MORE RADIOACTIVE IODINE

Seven days after the operation half of the 25 metal clips were taken out by the practice nurse at my GP surgery, and the rest of them the following day. I collected a sick certificate to send to my employer, and awaited a follow up appointment with the surgeon on December 22nd to find out the results of the biopsies.

The pain was still quite raw even nearly three weeks later when I saw the surgeon again. Unfortunately the follow up appointment proved to be rather disappointing. No results from the biopsies were available, and so I realised I had to spend Christmas in limbo, not knowing if I now had an aggressive form of cancer or not. The surgeon assured me that he would write to me as soon as he received the results. On a happier note, he was pleased at how well I had come through the operation, and how well the scar on the right side was healing (I now had the full 'necklace' from ear to ear).

I mentioned my two-tone, breathy voice. He passed the hated camera up my right nostril again, and down the back of my throat. After listening to me counting from one to ten, he could see that the one working vocal cord I possessed was still working, but had moved away slightly from the paralysed one, possibly he thought due to the endotracheal tube being in place for such a long time. He said he would refer me for speech therapy, but seemed confident that my voice would recover in time. I was impatient to be well again. Phil told me to be a *patient* patient.

I could not be bothered much with Christmas preparations. Phil put 6,000 fairy lights in the garden, which cheered me up with their beauty (they won the village Christmas Lights Competition!), but I had no desire to put up a tree or decorations inside the house. I did cook a turkey on Christmas Eve to take to Lee and Sarah's the following day, and we went to a carol service with Matt and Anna in the evening at the church they had been married in, but that was about all I felt like doing.

Sarah did us proud with a lovely dinner on Christmas Day, and there was a family meal at a local restaurant on Boxing Day, where we met Cousin Phillip and his partner who had travelled over from Saudi Arabia for the holidays. Unfortunately after Boxing Day I came down with the mother and father of all colds/flu bug, which took a week to shift, and removed totally what little voice I had. However, to make me feel better I started to notice that some of my novels (written under a pen name) were starting to sell quite well. I looked forward to seeing if the sales for 2015 would exceed those in 2014. It was a good start in January, as I managed to sell 108 books, as opposed to just 8 in January 2014. I also managed to attract the attention of a small publisher, who decided that he liked the book I was currently working on and wanted to publish it. He sent me a contract to look over and sign.

One of the best feelings in the sheworld when you're a bit down in the dumps is to have your hair cut and styled. I actually managed to drive myself to my hairdressers in Bury St Edmunds on 8th January, and it was wonderful to have my independence back and not be reliant on Phil to drive me about. The post-op pain was receding now, and people were telling me that my voice definitely sounded stronger when I spoke to them on the phone.

On returning from the hairdressers there was a message on the answerphone from my oncologist's secretary to tell me I needed to make an appointment to see the oncologist to obtain the results from the biopsies, which were now available. My heart immediately did a back flip of fear. I still had some grace with the insurance company before the New Year started in March, and so made an appointment to see her at the Cambridge Nuffield on 19th January. It was all hospitals and doctors; on the 12th January I was due to see the dermatologists at the department where I worked just to check on a few moles I had. I looked forward to popping in to the office and catching up on the gossip with my workmates.

On January 9th I was due for a bone scan to check that my osteopenia (due to having been over-medicated on Thyroxine) had not progressed to full-blown osteoporosis. I would be told my results at my appointment with the rheumatologist on February 15th. On January 12th Phil and I attended the Dermatology Department where I work to have some moles checked. I had already had a basal cell carcinoma removed three years before, but fortunately all the suspicious moles on my legs were found to be dermatofibromas. Phil had one mole on his wrist that the doctor wanted to remove, as he had no idea what it was.

With much trepidation I visited the oncologist on 19th January to get the results of the biopsies. She informed me that at least 15 nodes in my neck had been positive for papillary thyroid cancer, but reassured me that the cancer still seemed to be just a local recurrence, and that I was not terminal. She also told me that she had worked out a treatment plan; this would consist of more radioactive iodine back in the RAI suite at Addenbrooke's hospital, and then another scan to see if there had been any uptake. If there had not been, then

I would probably need guided external beam radiation as well. If none of these treatments worked, then a new drug, Sorafenib, was a possible option. However, this was only given as a last resort after I had exhausted all possible treatment options.

I looked up Sorafenib on the Internet; the drug had serious adverse side effects, and there was some question as to whether it actually improved overall survival at all. Marvellous! I also researched a list of the side effects:

<u>Common side-effects:</u>
- Rash
- Diarrhoea
- Fatigue

<u>Less common side-effects:</u>
- High blood pressure
- Hair loss (thinning or patchy hair loss)
- Nausea
- Itching
- Low white blood cell count (putting the patient at increased risk of infection)
- Poor appetite
- Vomiting
- Bleeding
- Increased amylase/lipase blood counts
- Low phosphorus level
- Constipation
- Shortness of breath
- Cough
- Numbness, tingling or pain in hands and feet
- Low platelet count

- Dry skin
- Abdominal pain
- Bone, muscle or joint pain
- Headache
- Weight loss

The date for my fourth dose of radioactive iodine was set for Monday 2nd March 2015. My heart sank at the prospect of more sore salivary glands, increased phlegm production at the back of my nose and throat, and possibly narrowing of the tear duct in my right eye necessitating a second DCR. The only good news for January was that my daughter-in-law Anna was due to give birth round about the 30th or 31st. Phil and I were on red alert to collect our grandson William and bring him back to ours for a few days. I mused on how strange it was that every time I had suffered a recurrence of this hateful disease in the past that needed treatment, I had also been presented with another grandchild at the same time. This one would be number four. As one door closes, another one opens......

The door opened on January 29th when I received a call at 3.30am from Matt to inform me that Anna's waters had broken and that she was 'definitely in labour'. I was instantly wide awake, jumping out of bed, getting dressed quickly, and searching for my car keys. By 4.45 I was picking up a very groggy William from his Mummy and Daddy, and bringing him home in my car. Phil was away on business for the week, and William and I spent a happy morning playing with his cars, and then visiting the Rosie Maternity Hospital in the afternoon to see new grandson Robert Anthony John Shepherd. Happier times!

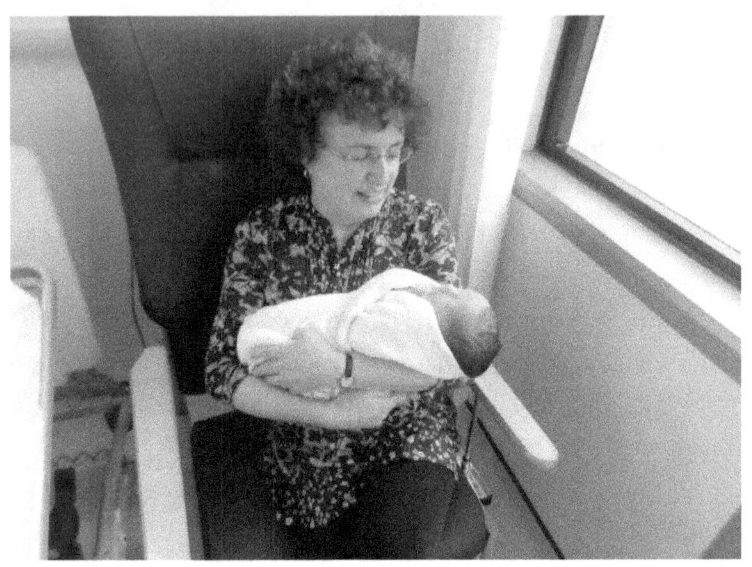

CHAPTER 43 – GIVING UP WORK

Meanwhile my voice had still not improved much since the operation in December, and the surgeon had referred me for voice therapy. I received the first appointment for voice exercises through the post, scheduled for February 6th 2015. I went along to the hospital where I work and saw the therapist, who showed me how to do diaphragmatic breathing and to use this in conjunction with structured exercises enabling the vocal cords to be pushed together. For one of the exercises I had to blow bubbles through a straw into a cup of water. I had always been given a disapproving look from my mother when I had carried out this action as a child, and it was quite strange to be doing this 40 years later! However, after a few weeks of doing these I could still feel no improvement to my voice.

On February 16th I began the low-iodine diet in preparation for more RAI treatment. It was a boring fortnight with no fish, nothing containing any form of soya, and nothing with additive E127 in. Phil decided he would make me some bread, as I could not find any that didn't contain soya flour. We borrowed a bread maker from Anna's mother, and Phil slowly became very proficient at knocking up loaves. I would have rather gone without any bread at all than stand in the kitchen kneading and rolling out dough, but Phil insisted that he wanted to do it. The result was thick slices of warm heavenly-smelling bread without any soya or preservatives, and I will be forever grateful that he took the time to learn how to use the machine.

I had been writing novels during my time off work, and was pleased to find a small publisher in February who wanted to publish my eighth novel (written under a pen-name). I duly signed a contract, and looked forward to publication in May. I also won a New Apple Book Award medal for one of my earlier novels, and I started to think about not going back to work at the hospital and try to make a living as an author. Sales had improved slowly, and there was nothing I wanted more than to sit at home all day and write. I had a sick certificate until the end of March, and decided to broach the subject with Phil. He was all for it, but at the last minute I decided to check with my manager first to see if there were any grade 3 secretarial jobs available where I did not have to answer the telephone. She sent an email to let me know she was 'working on it'.

Monday morning March 2nd saw me once again walking up to Ward A5 in Addenbrooke's hospital for my fourth dose of RAI treatment. This time there was no cheery Ann to bustle about getting me newspapers and extra pillows. She had either retired or had been made redundant. In fact nobody came into the room at all for the first 2 hours, and Phil and I wondered why I was asked to come in so early. As usual at 2.30 the physicist arrived, but this time brought a tiny capsule instead of the radioactive drink I had had three times previously. Progress had been made in the ensuing 10 years! All I had to do was to tip up the lead-lined box and let the capsule fall through a plastic screwed-on straw into my mouth. There was also no bottle of neutralising liquid that I needed to sprinkle down the loo as I had to do on previous occasions, and each room now had its own shower (bliss!). This time the hospital also made sure my low-iodine diet was adhered to (they had not done this before), but food was rather dry and the portions were meagre. I spent quite a lot of the time hungry, but Phil came to my rescue, got on his bike for a ride-out, and brought in some of his home-made bread from the freezer with some jam.

I stayed confined in the room until Wednesday morning, after being informed by the physicist measuring radiation levels with his rate meter, that my body had got rid of 95% of the radiation (the original dose was 5500 mega Becquerels). I had no side-effects, but wondered with hindsight when they would start arriving. I stocked up on barley sugars and cough candies just in case my salivary glands started becoming sore, and hoped against hope I did not have to undergo a new DCR on the right eye.

On the Thursday 5th March it was back to Addenbrooke's for my Gamma scan to see how much of the RAI my body had taken up, and where. The Gamma scanner was new and up-to-date, and it also took CT scans as well. I had a Gamma and a CT scan, and looked forward to receiving the results in April with some trepidation. Phil wasn't allowed to come in with me this time, as I had to wait in a room that was just solely for radioactive patients (one poor patient had a radioactive drip going into her arm!). The scans weren't as bad as an MRI, as this time my head did not have to be encased in a frame, and the machine was not noisy. I was informed that the Gamma scan would take 21 minutes, and the CT 11 minutes. I would not get the results until I saw the oncologist again on 20th April.

Meanwhile there was a check-up with the surgeon. I went to see him at the Bury BMI on 16th March. He told me he had taken out 47 nodes, 15 of which were cancerous. I mentioned my lack of a voice, and after looking at my vocal cords with the camera he reassured me that he could strengthen it with a thyroplasty operation. However, he did not want to do anything until August, to see if the voice came back on its own. After a meeting at work with my manager, it was agreed I could stay on extended sick leave until the end of May. I was in two minds whether to give up work altogether. The job was pressurised and stressful, and I was not looking forward to going back at all.

I eventually made the decision to stop work altogether a month later. The relief was overwhelming. I gave back my NHS badge and office key and felt no emotion whatsoever, even though I had been working at the hospital for 13 years. I did tell my manager that I might be back in 2016 as a bank secretary, but that I needed the rest of 2015 off to recover from all the treatments. My oncologist filled in a form and gave a good case for me to take my pension early.

The advantage of giving up work though meant that I could now concentrate fully on my writing. My fiction books were selling between 1 – 3 copies every day, the American publisher was on course to publish my latest novel in May, and after visiting the London Book Fair I might have U.K publishers interested in one of my novels regarding selling translation/foreign rights.

When I saw the oncologist on 20th April my voice was definitely stronger. She informed me that unfortunately my body had not taken up any of the RAI, and that I needed a CT scan (this time with contrast) on 11th May to determine whether I needed a 6-week course of external beam radiotherapy. My heart sank at the news. Why was my body so different from everyone else's? It made antibodies against thyroglobulin (which most people did not), and now it refused to take up any RAI. After 10 years of assaults on my body I was getting heartily sick of thyroid cancer.

CHAPTER 44 – FURTHER TREATMENT?

A few days after the CT scan with contrast I received a letter from my oncologist outlining everything that had taken place over the last few months. It did not make good reading, and brought home to me the fact that my life expectancy could possibly be shortened by the recent advancement of the disease. I have copied it word for word below:

'20th April 2015

Diagnosis:

(i)T4N1 papillary carcinoma of the thyroid June 2005 treated by total thyroidectomy followed by radioactive iodine.

(ii) Excision of left paratracheal mass and selective neck dissection August 2007.

(iii) Re-exploration of left thyroid bed and right selective neck dissection. Radioactive iodine given on 2/3/15. No evidence of uptake after 5.5 Gbq's of radioactive iodine administration.

It was a pleasure for me to see Glenda today in the clinic, who I am pleased to report is well. She tolerated her radioactive iodine with minimal side effects. She did have some hair loss, which may relate to the recombinant TSH injections. She is on thyroxine 100mcg per day with no adverse symptoms. I reminded her today that at the time of her operation the left thyroid surgical bed had recurrent papillary carcinoma which reached the resection margins, and her selective right neck dissection had 15 positive nodes between level 2 to level 4. There was evidence of focal extra nodal spread.

At the time of her radioiodine administration her TSH was 84 and there was some measurable thyroglobulin at 0.7 with 218 antithyroid globulin antibodies.

Because her thyroid cancer does not show evidence of radioiodine uptake, we would like her to consider the option of having external beam radiotherapy to her neck to try to prevent further local recurrence. This was following discussions in the thyroid cancer MDT.

I explained to Glenda today that radiotherapy treatment is often given to try and prevent further multiple surgical excisions being necessary. The reason we are considering this is we know that there is very likely to be residual microscopic disease in the neck. She understands that the radiotherapy does not bring any survival advantage, but is purely used to improve local control and has a good chance of doing this.

If she proceeded to treatment it would take place over six weeks, and would use intensity modulated and image-guided radiotherapy to a dose of 60 Gy in 30 fractions. The short term side-effects would include, but are not limited to, tiredness, skin soreness, intra oral mucositis, reduction in saliva, and change in taste. Many patients require a marked alteration in their diet and strong analgesia. It can occasionally affect swallowing. In the long term the risks associated with this treatment are small. There is a risk of further problems with swallowing, and sometimes oesophageal dilatation is necessary after treatment. There will be low risk of any harm to any important structures such as the spinal cord and brain stem, as these will be kept within a safe tolerance.

Before embarking on any treatment I think it would be helpful to have a restaging CT scan using IV contrast, and I have agreed to see Glenda back following the result of this investigation. She will spend some time thinking about whether she would like to proceed with radiotherapy.'

Wonderful. I did not need any time to think about it. I DIDN'T WANT IT! Not being able to swallow was not high on my list of pleasurable sensations. I became depressed, and decided to wait and see what the results of the scan showed. I told Phil that if the scan showed no cancer cells, then I was not going to have the treatment.

Meanwhile son Lee and daughter-in-law Sarah were at last able to obtain a mortgage and move into a 3-bed semi after an insurance policy I had been paying for 15 years finally matured and I was able to give them the deposit. I was happy to give the £10,000 away to them; by the sound of it I would have no need of the money anyway if my life was going to be cut short. They moved into their new home on 24th April 2015. At least two people were happy; Phil and I were not, but I kept the worst of it from them at the time.

I was beginning to hate living with thyroid cancer. The waiting was the worst; you wait for treatment, you wait for the scan appointment, and then you wait to see the consultant to find out if the treatment has worked and whether your life is to be shortened or not. Why can't they bloody well phone beforehand if the scan is okay and tell you not to worry? I was dreading the appointment with my oncologist on 11th May 2015 to obtain the CT scan result. However, I was pleasantly surprised to find that no evidence of any lumps could be seen. I immediately told her that I did not want the External Beam Radiotherapy treatment due to the serious side-effects it would cause. I asked her if she would want the treatment if she were in my shoes, but she did not answer! We agreed that I would have 3-monthly ultrasound scans instead, and that I would have the option of having the treatment if anything showed on the ultrasounds in the future. I also had to increase my thyroxine dose to 100mcg every day + 2 x 25mcg per week. I was happy at this, because I did wonder if the previous reduction in thyroxine had caused the thyroid stimulating hormone to become unsuppressed, causing remission to cease.

A friend at the British Thyroid Foundation put me in touch with a media representative from a drug company who were launching a new drug, Lenvima, for patients for differentiated thyroid cancer. Apparently the manufacturers were interested in patients like me whose thyroid cancer did not respond to radioactive iodine. The rep asked if I was willing to take part in a radio show to help with the launch, and I agreed. She phoned me at home on 13th May to ask about my cancer treatment and to make sure I would be willing to travel to a studio in central London one day in the near future to talk about my cancer journey. I agreed again. Expenses would be paid, and if the radio show did not eventually materialise, she said I could be involved in other launch promotions. I waited with excitement for the next phone call to confirm just how I would be taking part.

My 'fame' was spreading. In June the previous year I had been one of four patients filmed for the British Thyroid Foundation. A cameraman came to my house in June 2014 and spent a few hours filming me talking about thyroid cancer and how I coped with it. I hated to see how old I looked compared to the other three sufferers when the short 5-minute film was finally released in late 2014! I have added the link to it below. I was allowed to promote my books on the film too, and enjoyed a brief flurry in sales:

https://www.youtube.com/watch?v=6kSneADQedM

The clinic letter arrived to summarise my latest appointment with the oncologist. It was addressed to the surgeon who performed my neck dissections, and copied to myself and my GP:

'It was a pleasure for me to see Glenda today (11.05) in my clinic. She continues on thyroxine 125mcg one day a week and 100 mcg for the rest of the week (the oncologist had actually emailed me to take 2 x 125mcg before I received the letter). *As you know you recently resected her recurrent thyroid carcinoma and our MDT discussion was to consider proceeding on to external beam to the thyroid bed. She has had CT neck*

and thorax undertaken which did not show any significant problem in the thyroid bed, and no cervical, supraclavicular or other lymph nodes. There are some small lung nodules which have been noted previously.

I had a long discussion with Glenda today about the role of external beam radiation in terms of local control. At present she would like to continue with an observation policy. I have therefore booked for her to have an ultrasound in three months' time; this will be before your next planned appointment to see her on 03.08.2015. I have made a further follow-up appointment on 09.11.2015 at 11.15 for Glenda to see me. In the interim I have also agreed I will send her some more detailed information on external beam radiotherapy, and I will also endeavour to find a patient who might be able to discuss their experience with her.'

CHAPTER 45 – FULL-TIME AUTHOR

The radio show did not seem to be materialising, but meanwhile there was the usual Isle of Wight festival to enjoy and take my mind off my troubles. Phil and I made the journey over to the Island on Friday 12th June, staying in the same Shanklin hotel as the previous year. We were lucky to only have rain on the Friday evening this time, and enjoyed the likes of Paolo Nutini, The High Kings, The Prodigy, and best of all Fleetwood Mac, who headlined on the last night. I managed the walking around okay, and even tried a little of the Tennyson Trail at Freshwater on the Monday before we came home, but by then my legs were complaining.

When we got back I decided I'd like to visit Matthew Manning again, a spiritual healer. I had previously seen him several years before when he lived in Lavenham, Suffolk. When I got in touch with his secretary I was dismayed to find that he now worked in Ashburton, Devon, over 200 miles away. Phil, nonetheless, was willing to drive me there and back, and although he viewed spiritual healing with a healthy dose of suspicion he was happy to let me do my thing. I made two appointments for healing for Monday 29th June, and booked us a cheap bed and breakfast opposite the health clinic where the healing was to take place.

Ashburton is a quaint, pretty little town. We found The Haven

Health Clinic at 24 West Street, and I was pleased to discover that Matthew still remembered me. The two half an hour sessions took place and he seemed assured that 'it would keep the men in white coats away'. I sincerely hoped he was right. He informed me that he would have also sought out other alternative therapies as I was doing before considering the external beam radiotherapy, as he told me that once that particular treatment had been carried out, then that option would be exhausted. I nodded in agreement. He was happy to treat me again whenever I wished.

I had changed my mind regarding my American publisher, and decided to stay self-published. I preferred to have full control over the pricing of my novels, and contacted him to break the news. Fortunately he was agreeable. During the month of June I sold 143 novels, a bumper month! July was even better, with 160 novels sold.

A friend from my schooldays came to stay overnight in June whilst Phil was in the USA on business. We had a lovely time catching up and visiting Newmarket races, where unfortunately I lost all my bets. She was worried about her husband, who was also being monitored for a recurrence of cancer. It seemed that I and her husband had lots in common. We arranged to meet up again in October, but this time Phil and I would travel to visit them.

Towards the end of July I had a letter from the Pensions' Agency. It seemed that my application for ill-health retirement had been accepted. I had officially given up work on 21st June 2015, but in reality had not been working as a medical secretary since 3rd December 2014. I was now a full-time self-employed author! I was soon given details of my occupational pension benefits and lump sum, which I received in August 2015. The lump sum was immediately put away to cover most of the cost of central heating to our house, which would be installed in May 2016.

Only too soon 28th July came around and it was time once again to travel to Addenbrooke's for another ultrasound scan. Phil decided he wanted to drive me there this time, I suppose to be around in case the news was bad. However, I was getting somehow used to the Grim Reaper sitting on my shoulder. I had every hope and all fingers crossed that nothing would show up and that I would not need the external beam radiation. The side-effects were horrendous, and I knew I would become very sick indeed.

It was the same doctor in the scanning room who I saw before. I think he remembered me too, which was a bonus. He put some gel on my neck and within a few minutes he gave me the good news that he could not see anything in my neck that should not be there. I gave a huge sigh of relief and looked at Phil, who was grinning from ear to ear. Thank goodness we would not need to cancel our holiday to Menorca on 18th September, or cancel the writer's course I had booked at York University or our weekend with friends in Cheltenham in October. I was free to enjoy the rest of the summer before another scan at the end of October. I also decided to book another appointment with Matthew Manning, as his clinic was further along the M5 from our friends in Cheltenham, and was granted an appointment for Monday 12th October.

At the beginning of August I had a follow up appointment with the ENT surgeon. He slid the camera up my right nostril and down the back of my throat, and confirmed that the one working vocal cord was in a slightly better position. My voice was slightly stronger at last, and I asked him if he could do anything to make it even stronger. He said that he could, but it might leave me short of breath. I decided there and then not to have any further procedures done on my voice, and he discharged me but agreed to refer me to the ophthalmologist I saw in 2009 as my right eye was beginning to water with the effects of the radiation I had had in March.

The ophthalmologist washed out my right tear duct, which he

thought might be slightly blocked as he had to apply a firm pressure for me to be able to taste the saline at the back of my throat. He said that he would refer me for a Nuclear Medicine dacryoscintigram of the lacrimal duct. Radioactive eye drops would be put in my eyes, and then a succession of x-rays would be taken over about an hour or so. I was worried about the amount of radiation I had had over the year, but I checked with the oncologist who said the eye drops would only contain a low amount of radiation. I was booked in for this procedure on 21st October at Addenbrooke's, which coincided quite nicely with another ultrasound of the neck.

Meanwhile there was Menorca to enjoy. Phil and I flew out from Stansted airport on 18th September for a week at the resort of Arenal d'en Castell. Fortunately it wasn't too hot, and we swam in a warm clear sea, went on a powerboat ride and also a boat ride around Mahon harbour, visited the Caves of Xoroi and Binibeca (the picturesque 'sugar cube' village), and watched the dancing horse show at Cala Galdana. All in all it was a very enjoyable holiday. The hotel catered for only couples, so there were no screaming children around the pool. There's something about not wanting to spend your holiday with other people's children once your own have grown up isn't there?

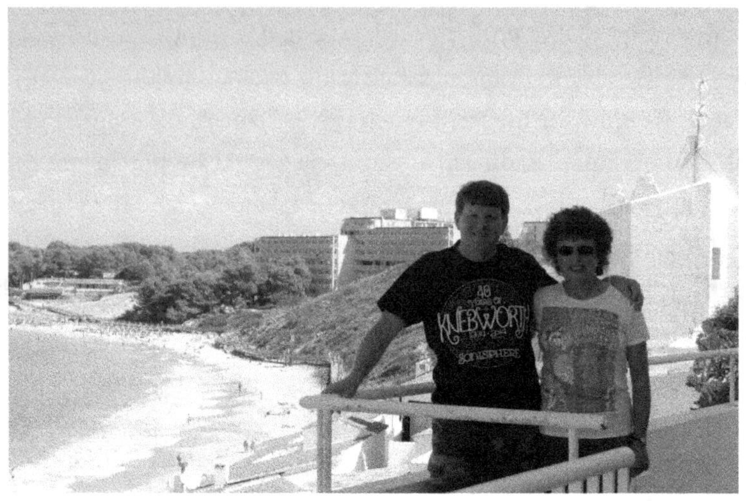

Phil and I at the resort of Arenal d'en Castell in Menorca.

Back home again I decided to cancel the dacryoscintigram, as I was worried about the cumulative effect of more radiation to my head. I decided just to go for another DCR operation to my right eye instead, which was booked for 7th January 2016. I asked the secretary regarding not being intubated, and back came the reply that the anaesthetist could use a laryngeal mask instead, so that no tubes touched my voice box. I was relieved about this, as my voice still hadn't returned properly from the neck dissection in December 2014. It was weaker than it was before, but I reasoned that I would just have to live with it.

We had a lovely weekend away on 10th and 11th October, seeing friends who live in Winchcombe, Gloucestershire. We were tourists for the weekend and enjoyed visiting Sudeley Castle, home of Catherine Parr, amongst others. We dined out at the Royal Oak in Gretton, and also celebrated our 35th wedding anniversary on 11th October. I was pleased to receive a jade necklace from Phil, and bought him an engraved paperweight to mark the occasion.

On Monday 12th October we drove further along the M5 to The

Haven Health Clinic in Ashburton so that I could see Matthew Manning for another healing session. Funnily enough, later on after the healing took place I actually slept all night without waking up, which is something I had not done since I was a teenager! Matthew also told me he would help with marketing my books by advertising them on his Facebook page. Everything was going well.

CHAPTER 46 – MATT IS 30!

On 21ST October 2015 it was time to trundle along the A14 again to Addenbrooke's for another ultrasound scan. I was suffering with a horrible throat infection and cold. When my name was called out I was disappointed to see that it wasn't the usual radiologist performing the scan who I and the oncologist had complete faith in. This time the doctor looked younger than my sons. I had a gut feeling that this scan would not go well.

It didn't. The doctor told me the left side was fine, but there was an enlarged lymph node on the right side which had not been there on the previous scan, but that it didn't look like thyroid tissue. I asked him if my germ would have had anything to do with it, and he said it was a possibility. I would have to wait for the Wednesday morning multi-disciplinary meeting on October 28th between my oncologist, neck surgeon and the radiologists to get a better diagnosis.

My heart was in my boots once again imagining the worst as the meeting drew nearer. What didn't help was Mum asking me to book a pre-paid funeral for her. So there was I sitting in the undertaker's parlour on the Monday morning organising my 91 year old mother's funeral, and all the time thinking my own might well be coming before hers. However, my own demise was fortunately to be put on hold, as I received an email from my oncologist on my birthday to say that the consensus of opinion at the meeting was that I just needed another ultrasound in 3 – 6 months' time. They could see 2 tiny nodes on the right side of the neck, but they were too small to biopsy, and at the moment were too difficult to diagnose. What it did mean though, was the fact that I'd have this uncertainty hanging over my head all over Christmas and into the New Year.

Matt's 30th birthday party was looming. I had organised a disco and catering in our village hall for November 21st, and the party helped to take my mind off my troubles. It was nice to see family and friends who despite the terrible weather (and even a power cut that morning due to strong winds) had made the effort to come along. Most of Matt's friends had small children, and the hall had a small ante-room where I set up some toys usually played with by the village Mother & Toddlers' group. For the adults there was a bar and dancing, and the evening went with a swing.

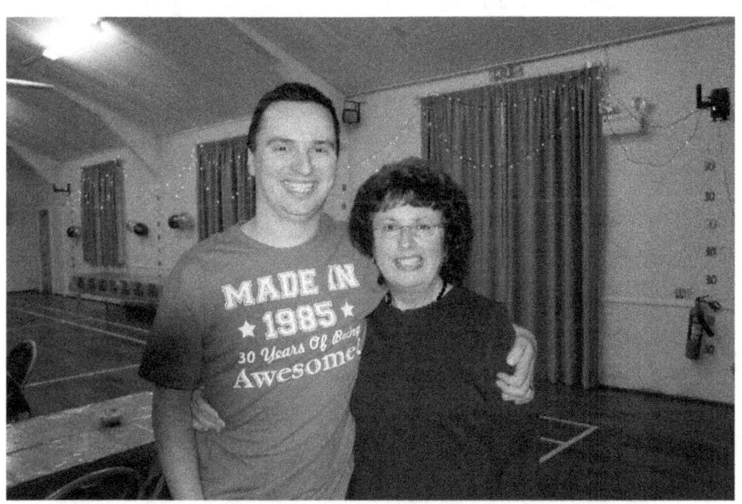

Matt and I at the start of his 30th birthday party 21/11/15

On Christmas Day I had no time to think about what might be growing in my neck. During the morning we visited Mum, who for the first time on the big day was refusing to leave her flat. We joined my cousin Phillip and stayed with her for a couple of hours, and then

Phil and I went to see Lee and Sarah and our two granddaughters to exchange presents. After that it was time to visit Matt and Anna and their two boys at Ipswich, where they were staying overnight with Anna's parents. Being busy was probably the best thing for me, and I was able to put maudlin thoughts to the back of my mind.

On New Year's Eve Phil and I stayed at a flat in London's Covent Garden which we had booked up eleven months previously! We strolled around the corner to the Strand Palace Hotel for a delicious carvery dinner, and then walked for an hour through the London streets thronging with people to Tower Hill Pier to catch one of the tourist boats up to Westminster in order to watch the fireworks erupting from the London Eye. The weather was kind to us, and Big Ben's chimes at midnight heralded the old year out and the new one in. As I watched the fireworks sparkle and fizzle I wondered what 2016 held in store for me.

CHAPTER 47 – ANOTHER DCR OPERATION

I did not have long to wait. On 5th January 2016 I had a bone density scan performed at the BMI hospital at Bury St Edmunds, ready for my appointment with the rheumatologist in February. On 7th January it was time to undergo another operation. I had managed to evade the operating theatre for the whole of 2015, but my watery right eye now needed treatment with a dacryocystorhinostomy (DCR) before I started to have the constant infections that had besieged my left eye back in 2009. I wanted to get the op over with in case I needed more radiation treatment in February. This time the operation would be done endoscopically from the inside of my nose, as I have a deviated septum allowing more room for the surgeon to work on the right side. There would be no scar.

It was a ride of death to the Spire Lea hospital. Persistent rain had flooded the roads, and walls of water from passing lorries washed over the car as we drove along the A14. Nobody was more relieved than I was when we turned off the motorway and pulled up outside the Spire Lea.

I was quite disappointed at being shown to a small cubicle housing a bed, cabinet, and one chair for Phil in a busy day surgery unit instead of having the usual room of my own. Because I was a short stay patient, this time I would not be staying overnight on the ward.

Luckily the surgeon's list was not very long; only two patients and I was second. I'm usually always last on the surgical lists, as word gets around that I'm the 'tricky one' with the paralysed vocal cord. However, I was reassured by the anaesthetist who told me he would be using a laryngeal mask this time, so hopefully my voice would not disappear as it had done for most of 2015. I was wheeled to the anaesthetic room around 9.30am, where the anaesthetist put a cannula in my hand and told me to have 'pleasant dreams' as he shot me full of a liquid cosh that addicts all over the world are fighting each other to get at.

I woke up about an hour and a half later with a plug under my nose to catch drips of blood. Of course my heart rate and blood pressure were sky high as they usually are after operations, and I was kept on the recovery ward a bit longer than most patients are under the same circumstances. However, I was allowed to go home about 2pm, and feeling very delicate I was wheeled out to the car park by a nurse, with Phil following behind. I was told not to blow my nose for a week, or have any hot drinks. I was given Maxitrol eye drops and a nasal spray to be used for a month, and another appointment to see the surgeon for a follow up appointment a week later on 14th January. I was pleased to discover that thankfully what was left of my voice was still intact.

It was hell not being able to blow my nose. Both sides of my nose felt blocked, and it was difficult to eat and drink as I could only breathe through my mouth. Blood seeped down the right nostril for two days, and I ran out of the little pads the nurses gave me to soak it up. I didn't remember having such a blocked nose when the left side was done, although this had been performed from the outside, leaving a scar. However, after two weeks the procedure had been worth it, as my eye no longer watered all the time. The follow up appointment went well, and I just had to return on February 10th to have the stent taken out.

In preparation for my visits to the oncologist on 1st February for the results of my latest ultrasound scan, and the rheumatologist on 23rd February, I had a thyroid function blood test and a bone profile done beforehand. Results seemed good; the thyroid stimulating hormone was still suppressed at 0.04, and my bone profile was normal. My Vitamin D level had risen from 38 to 46, and so was almost normal (should be 50).

On January 25th 2016 it was time for another of my three-monthly ultrasound scans. In view of the two slightly enlarged nodes on the right side of my neck which they had found on the last scan, I was not feeling very optimistic as regards the outcome. On the drive to Addenbrooke's Hospital I chatted with Phil about how we were going to cope with a possible 6-week treatment of radiation. I mentioned that perhaps if I drove myself for as long as I was able to before side-effects set in, then Phil would only need to drive me there for maybe three of the six weeks. If I had the first appointment every morning and Phil worked an extra couple of hours at the end of the day, then perhaps his employers would not get too uptight about his late starts. Phil told me very firmly to wait and see what the scan showed first.

My heart felt as though it was going to leap out of my chest as I lay on the couch. This time a consultant radiologist whom I had never seen before undertook the procedure. To my utter delight he informed me that the two nodes on the right looked as though they had possibly shrunk, and that he could not see any sign of thyroid cancer anywhere in my neck. His words made my day, and I was so elated I forgot to visit the toilet on the way out and had to go back in! When I saw the oncologist for a follow up appointment a week later she reiterated what the radiologist had said, confirming my clear scan and lack of neck lumps when she felt around my neck. She did however say that I had a lot of 'tightening' in my neck. Yes, I could definitely feel the adhesions, but was told that nothing could be done about them.

I asked the oncologist about proton beam radiotherapy, as I had heard a lot about it. She said it was not suitable for thyroid cancer as it is a targeted treatment suitable for spine tumours, but with the neck the radiation needs to be widespread. I also asked her whether my adhesions were to blame for muscle pain at the tops of my arms, but she did not know. I had a blood test for thyroglobulin, and she told me that I could leave it 6 months instead of 3 months now before I needed another ultrasound scan and follow up. This was confirmed in her clinic letter below:

It was a pleasure to see Glenda today (01/02/16) in my clinic, who is on 100mcg of thyroxine five days per week and 125mcg two days per week. She feels her energy levels are satisfactory, although does acknowledge she is a bit more tired than previously. She gets occasional palpitations, but these are not causing major concern. Her most recent T4 is 26.7, with a T3 of 4.5 and a TSH of 0.04.

On examination today she looked very well, and there was no sign of recurrence in her neck. She had an ultrasound performed on 25th January and this has shown that the previously noted small nodules medial to the right common carotid artery now measure 4 x 3mm, which is smaller than previously reported.

I have arranged to see Glenda again in August, and will book an ultrasound prior to this visit. I have also checked her serum thyroglobulin, and will repeat all of the bloods at her next visit.

With written confirmation of the shrinking nodules, I decided to arrange another visit to healer Matthew Manning, and contacted his secretary as soon as I returned home. She gave me an appointment for 10am on 4th April, and so I let our friends in Winchcombe know that we would be popping in to see them on Sunday April 3rd. Now all I needed to do was to have the stent in my eye removed on January

10th, and see the rheumatologist at the end of February.

Having a good result fills one with much hope for the future. I decided that now I could book up a couple of hotels for trips we were thinking about, and I also paid the deposit on a week's holiday in the Isle of Wight. We would attend the music festival in June, and then have a few days over to laze on the beach or visit our favourite tourist attractions. Three days after receiving the good result we 'pushed the boat out' again and booked up a cruise for our 60th birthdays which would stop in New Orleans at Mardi Gras. We would fly out to Miami on February 19th 2017, and spend 2 weeks cruising, stopping at Georgetown, Grand Cayman, Puerto Costa Maya, Mexico, and Cozumel as well as 3 days in New Orleans. I refused to think about having to cancel it in order to receive external beam radiotherapy.

Although it looked good for me, our ten year old granddaughter Sophie was not progressing well. It was originally thought she had Woolf-Parkinson-White Syndrome, but heart scans and tests showed that this was not the case. A re-surgence of her strange attacks were taking place whereby her heart would race, her lips would turn blue, and on bad attacks she could not feel her legs. She was given beta blockers and an appointment for the Brompton Heart Hospital in March. The beta blockers made her tired and slow. I told my daughter-in-law that I was available to accompany her for Sophie's appointment now that I knew I didn't have to undergo any treatment for the time being. I did wonder if the attacks were perhaps due to a food intolerance, as my heart usually produced ectopic beats if I ate anything sweet, but my daughter-in-law assured me that Sophie had passed food allergy tests with flying colours. It also occurred to me to wonder whether Sophie possibly had an overactive thyroid, but decided to wait until she had been to the Brompton. As a grandmother I had learned that unfortunately I had to take a back seat and keep my opinions to myself!

However, Sophie's strange heart episodes were passed off by the consultant at the Brompton as something she would probably grow out of. She was given a 14 day heart monitor to wear, much to her disgust, but thankfully the consultant did not seem too worried. He took her off the beta blockers, and told my son and daughter-in-law that she should not have been put on them in the first place! It just confirmed to me that you could never get two doctors to agree on anything.

CHAPTER 48 – A NEEDLE BIOPSY

The stent in my right eye came out much easier than on the left side in 2009. However, the result wasn't as good as the left side at first, which had been an external DCR (the operation on my right eye had been an internal DCR, as the surgeon had told me that techniques had moved on since 2009). On the day following the removal my eye was still red and watery, although I seemed to have caught a germ. Blowing my nose felt most peculiar; air rushed across my eye, and the whole eye filled up with water. I found out that the best way to blow my nose and avoid these effects was to keep both eyes shut.

The germ intensified. My throat was sore, I had chills and muscle aches, and on the Monday following my stent removal I had to go to A&E as both eyes were blood red and filled with pus. I felt and looked terrible. I was given Chloramphenicol ointment 1% and told to put it in both eyes 4 times per day. The GP eventually gave me Clarithromycin antibiotics after 9 days had passed and I still did not feel recovered. The two antibiotics cleared up the sore throat and eye infection, and 6 weeks after the surgery my right eye seemed to have improved. The droopy eyelid had resolved, and both eyes were now a normal colour and non-watery. However, the right eye still felt sore sometimes in the mornings, and looked a little bloodshot first thing. I made a mental note to inform the surgeon if the problem had not resolved by the time I had my follow up appointment in May.

The last hospital appointment for a while occurred on February 23rd, when I visited the hospital where I used to work for an NHS appointment with the rheumatologist. I saw a new consultant this time, who was pleased with my bone scan and bone profile, and said that I did not need to come back for another bone scan and follow up appointment until February 2018. She also told me to take less or no calcium, as this had been shown in new research to cause heart problems. This was in direct conflict with the advice I had been given previously! The consultant informed me that vitamin D was more important for my bones than calcium. Mulling over her advice I decided to take less calcium, and reduced my Calcichew tablets to one a day rather than two. I also bought some low-dose over-the-counter vitamin D tablets, fervently hoping they would not cause an increase in ectopic heart beats, as a high dose had done some years previously.

After a few weeks I decided to stop the Calcichew altogether, and instead of the vitamin D tablets (which did in fact cause an increase in ectopic beats) I took a multi-vitamin specially formulated for women of 50+ years, which had a lower dose of vitamin D added. I now had 6 clear months without having to see any doctor, apart from the follow up with the eye surgeon in May, which I could cancel if it was not needed.

Unfortunately I soon found the 6 clear months turned out to be a trifle premature, as mid-March I was back for an emergency appointment with the ENT surgeon at the Nuffield hospital in Cambridge to investigate a lump I'd had on the left side of my neck for about 3 weeks. My opinion was either of a swollen salivary gland, or a lymph node that was still up from the germ in February, but I needed peace of mind. The surgeon arranged for an ultrasound and possible needle biopsy to be performed the following day. He said the lump, which was pulsating, was too low to be a salivary gland but might be a 'tortuous artery'. However, he like me needed to know that any tumours had not returned.

With all the surgery I'd had in the past, I'd never undergone a needle biopsy. The experience was less than pleasant, and at one time I knew how people felt who were being strangled. Under ultrasound the radiologist could see the lump was an enlarged lymph node which was sitting on top of an artery, hence the pulsing. He took 3 samples after injecting the side of my neck with local anaesthetic, and once again I waited on tenterhooks until I found out the result. The bruising was spectacular, and looked as though I had an industrial hickey.

The waiting is terrible. Anybody who has been through this will know what I mean. In the still of the night you can't sleep and think the worst. I started to imagine more external beam radiotherapy, mouth ulcers, hair loss, not being able to swallow, and a neck full of cancer again. After a week the lump had reduced in size somewhat, but I couldn't stand the waiting anymore and sent an email to my surgeon, who replied with this email on Easter Saturday:

'Good news, the biopsies have all come back as reactive, i.e no cancer seen. It would be good to see that the nodes shrink down however, so it would probably be best for you to make an appointment to see me in about a month if possible.'

I dutifully turned up for my appointment on 5th May, but all the surgeon could feel was the carotid artery on the left side of my neck. I'd undergone all that trauma for nothing, although Phil disagreed. He said I now had peace of mind, which I didn't have before.

The follow up appointment with the eye surgeon in June gave me reassurance that the new drain in the right eye was working fine. However, ongoing blepharitis, a poor quality tear film, and conjunctival chalasis (similar to dry eyes but with some pain as well) ensured that for the immediate future I would still be suffering with an intermittent watery right eye. He announced in the roundabout way that all doctors have that there wasn't much more he could do for me, and that I would have to live with it.

CHAPTER 49 – HOME IMPROVEMENTS

Phil and I had decided that 2016 was the year in which we made our home more saleable, ready for putting on the market when we were ready to downsize. To start this particular ball rolling we waited for Spring to arrive and then arranged for a plasterer to start working on skimming the downstairs walls ready for painting, and then for a local heating company to finally install central heating, 75 years after the house was built! I used my lump sum from my pension to take care of the central heating bill, and I think we must have been the only house in the road that had held out on installing central heating for so long. Being over-medicated on thyroxine ensures that you do not need much heat, and Phil prefers a cooler house too. The upheaval of refurbishment was something I would not wish upon anybody. The reception rooms had to be stripped back to the bare walls for the plasterer, and Calor Gas hired a mechanical excavator in order to dig a 6ft hole in our front garden for the underground gas tank. The neighbours had free entertainment while the low-loader parked outside in the road and a crane moved the tank from the low-loader into the hole.

In-between the tank being fitted and the workmen from the central heating company arriving and invading every corner of our house, there was the Isle of Wight Festival to enjoy. The weather was quite kind to us this year, and the site did not turn into a mudbath. Headliners Queen with Adam Lambert were the main attraction, with The Who next in line. I consider that all the time I can walk up to the site and make my way around the many stalls and attractions, then I'm still well enough. I also try and walk part of the Tennyson Trail at Freshwater Bay the day after the festival has ended. A few years back I could make it as far as the monument, but now I'm happy if I can just get halfway with the aid of my walking poles. The 5 days at the Isle of Wight was our main holiday in 2016, as we decided to save for a cruise to New Orleans' Mardi Gras in February 2017 to celebrate our forthcoming 60th birthdays.

Soon after the festival it was time for our 1940's house to become catapulted into the modern age. Carpets and floorboards were taken up everywhere, workmen hammered, drilled and soldered all day for over a week. Furniture had to be moved out into the garage, which unfortunately flooded during a very non-British storm on 20th July that resembled a tropical monsoon. Some of our furniture was soaked, which only added to the nightmare, and so Phil had to cart it all back into the living room. I prayed for peace and quiet again, but this took nearly two weeks to achieve.

As well as *our* household being disrupted, it was also time for my 92 year old mother to move into very sheltered housing to receive the extra care she needed as she was very frail and had started to fall more often. Within a week of our central heating being installed, poor old Mum was uprooted from her council flat. She had been against the change for some time, but once she had moved in she could see that it was a much better flat, and it had more space for her to walk around in. She and I felt happier that there were carers on duty at night in case of an emergency, and she even had a spare bedroom for friends to stay in. Phil set up her keyboard/organ in the spare room, and she called it her 'music room'.

On August 3rd it was time for me to make another trip to Addenbrooke's hospital for a follow up ultrasound scan. It's always a worrying time before the scan, and I do not usually sleep well the previous night. However, I was pleased to be informed that that scan was clear. I was sent the date for my next scan, which I found out was only a week before we set off on our cruise. Just to help the next result along I booked another session of healing with Matthew Manning down at his clinic in Devon.

My poor unfortunate mother had only been in her flat 2 and a half months when she suffered a mini-stroke. I was with her on the Saturday morning of 15th October when she complained of a loss of vision in one eye. She began slurring her words, and her mouth drooped down temporarily on one side. I called in the senior carer, who confirmed that Mum was not herself. She called the ambulance, and Mum was taken off to hospital. She was seen almost straight away in A&E, and within a short space of time was ensconced in the stroke ward. The next day was quite a shock for me, as when I visited she was talking 19 to the dozen, but none of it was making any sense. The doctors wanted to do an MRI scan, but I knew that Mum would not be able to lie still inside a scanner for 20 minutes. A CT scan of her head had shown nothing untoward, but I was afraid I had lost the mother I knew for good, and wept bitterly on the way home.

However, she had recovered slightly when I visited the next day. She was talking more coherently and had even lain still inside the MRI scanner for a head scan, the results of which showed no sign of a stroke. The doctors began treating her for a urine infection, but she was becoming weaker and struggled to stand up without help. She was pumped full of antibiotics and recovered well from the infection after a week in hospital, but the mini stroke had taken its toll. Back at home she was no longer interested in doing her daily crossword, and struggled to write anything. All she wanted to do was die, and staying alive now held no joy for her. She sat in her armchair and stared into space, no longer caring if her catheter bag was emptied by the carers or not. It was heart-breaking, especially when her brother, my Uncle Harry, also moved nearer to death with congestive cardiac failure and melanoma metastases. I took over everything, from paying all Mum's bills to even making up her shopping list. She was no longer the mother I had grown up with. Within a few more weeks her legs began to swell horribly with serous fluid. The doctor put her on Frusemide water tablets, and the district nurses came and went with depressing regularity to dress her watery legs. The swelling in her legs improved, but she became increasingly frail and could not walk at all without falling over, and after only 5 months in her new sheltered housing flat she was permanently bedridden. A nasty pressure sore began to develop on her back, because she could not lie in any other position other than on her back.

***

Phil and I tentatively began to look for a retirement property ourselves. We had our house valued, and found to our surprise it was worth £250,000. We had paid £69,000 for it back in 1991, and I traipsed around several estate agencies to see what was on offer. When we looked at retirement flats for the over 55's, we were quite disappointed to discover that we would be living in a complex similar to my mother's sheltered housing. Residents looked as though they had been 55 quite some time ago, and the flats were too tiny for the pair of us. Bike sheds were full of mobility scooters, much to Phil's disgust. We came to the conclusion quite separately that we would never be able to get away from each other unless we lived in separate flats! After looking around several more properties, we discovered that the nearer a property was to Bury St. Edmunds town centre, the more money it cost. Unfortunately we could find nothing better than we already had, and so made a joint decision to stay where we were for a few more years until we really *did* need the retirement flat.

242

CHAPTER 50 - COLONOSCOPY

I spent a pleasant 59th birthday down at the O2 concert arena in Greenwich with Phil to see the rock band Bad Company (I was glad I did, as guitarist Mick Ralphs suffered a stroke soon after the concert). We stayed overnight, and the next day we decided to take a 'flight' on the Emirates air-line (the U.K's first urban cable car) stretching over the Thames from Greenwich to the Royal Victoria Docks on the other side.

After the flight we walked along the Embankment enjoying the late autumn sunshine and the sight of many strangely dressed people gathered nearby for some type of science fiction convention. We stopped off in a café for a green tea, and I ate a banana and chuckled at the sights I could see out of the café's window.

As we left the café and walked further along to where the main convention was taking place, I was suddenly gripped with very strong and unpleasant pains in my abdomen. Soon after this I had a terrible urge to find a toilet. I looked around desperately. The convention was taking place outside a Novotel, and ignoring the sci-fi fans milling about and posing, I ran towards the hotel's foyer and tried not to sound too desperate as I asked for directions to a toilet. As soon as I came back outside again I told Phil that I wanted to go back to the car. We queued up at the Emirates air-line again, but I had another terrible urge and we had to find another toilet in a hurry in a café nearby.

I had never experienced anything like this before. I didn't have an upset stomach, and the situation had been quite distressing. I assumed the problem would eventually resolve, but after a couple of weeks it had not, and I was getting IBS-type symptoms of alternating constipation and diarrhoea. I visited the GP, who felt my abdomen and carried out one of those unpleasant PR examinations, but she could not find anything wrong. She referred me to a colorectal surgeon at the Nuffield Hospital, Cambridge. By then, a month later, the situation was getting somewhat better. He carried out the same tests, but had similarly unremarkable results, and so booked me for an abdominal ultrasound (again, nothing remarkable found) and a colonoscopy to investigate further. I was horrified to find out the colonoscopy involved taking a number of senna tablets and an industrial turbo-laxative, and not eating for 24 hours beforehand so that my bowels were completely empty for the procedure. I would then be lightly anaesthetised with Midazolam and Fentanyl. The colonoscopy was booked for January 12th 2017. Happy New Year…

***

Even on the Thames cruiser on New Year's Eve I was thinking about the colonoscopy. The fireworks blazed from the London Eye, and everyone around me was cheering, but I couldn't seem to join in with the bonhomie. I made all the right noises and smiled at the right moments, but all the time was worried in case the strong abdominal pains returned or that I had bowel cancer as well as thyroid cancer. Fortunately the pains did not return, but the colonoscopy hanging over my head made the start of 2017 rather a damp squib for me.

The low residue diet started on Tuesday 10th January, and carried on until lunchtime the following day, when I was not allowed to eat any more solid food until after the procedure. I filled up on white bread, white pasta and chicken, and the whole experience was quite constipating! However, I didn't have long to worry about that. At 2pm on Wednesday 11th January I returned from helping Mum with her lunch, and then down the little red lane went 4 senna tablets. I had lit the blue touch paper, but unfortunately couldn't stand back away from it all.

At 5pm I poured 8 fluid ounces of boiling water on the contents of the first sachet of Citramag powder. It fizzed up like the fireworks on New Year's Eve, and I lost some of it on the floor. Oh dear, no wonder the instructions said use a large jug! For the next half a sachet two hours later I used a saucepan. After that there was much gurgling down in the depths. I spent the rest of the evening and all night (13 hours in total) running backwards and forwards to the toilet until I was left with what seemed like a shell for a body, as it appeared that all my innards had been flushed away. Citramag is EVIL (I decided not to take the other half of the sachet that was recommended on Thursday morning)!

Thankfully the diarrhoea had stopped when it was time for Phil to drive me to the Nuffield Hospital in Cambridge for the procedure. It was a cold, murky January morning when we left, which didn't help to lift my spirits at all.

After an hour sitting around in room 23, a nurse appeared and informed me that I could put on the hated hospital gown that does up at the back. She also brought me a huge pair of paper knickers with an opening at the back (don't ask), which decided to start falling down as soon as I began to walk with the nurse to the operating theatre.

The surgeon greeted me, I lay down on my side on the trolley, and he put a cannula in my right arm. When he added some Midazolam sedation and Fentanyl painkiller I waited to feel drowsy, but unfortunately did not. I remember everything from the rather painful colonoscopy, although previously in the clinic he had told me that I would not be able to recall anything. I watched the insides of my bowels on the screen, shining with the aid of a lighty-up camera. They looked extremely clean! The surgeon told me that apart from a small polyp (which he removed for biopsy) and some pre-diverticular changes, there was nothing sinister to see. *Fankgawdferthat* as my old grandmother would have said.

I was taken into the recovery room, where I had a nice chat with one of the nurses, and then wheeled back to room 23. Phil told me afterwards that out of all the procedures and operations I'd had before, I looked the most awake this time. I had a nasty feeling that I hadn't been given much sedation at all.

We went home an hour later, and I slept like a log all night. Now, bowel cancer free, I was eager to enjoy our cruise to New Orleans for the Mardi Gras scheduled for February 18th.

CHAPTER 51 – NEW ORLEANS

Two more things marred my joy before we went away. My mum, now 92, had begun to deteriorate with a grade 4 pressure sore just before Christmas, and by the beginning of February she was hospitalised and on Social Services' list for a nursing home, which she was moved to just before we left for Heathrow, leaving us to begin the sad task of clearing out her flat. Her quality of life was poor, and the prognosis was bleak. She was given about three more months of life, but she implored me to go on holiday and have a good time. However, I knew I'd feel guilty for leaving her all the time I was away.

Another ultrasound scan on my neck performed on 31st January at Addenbrooke's hospital showed possible activity in the thyroid bed. The radiologist wasn't sure whether thyroid cancer was present, and stated that he would leave it to my oncologist to decide whether she wanted to do nothing and review with another scan in the near future, to request another biopsy, or to start 6 weeks of external beam radiotherapy. I would now have this bad news hanging over my head for the duration of our holiday. The New Year wasn't as full of joy as I'd hoped it would be.

I visited the oncologist on Friday 10th February. As I suspected, she confirmed the growth of a new nodule on the right of the thyroid bed, and was keen for the 6 weeks of external beam radiotherapy to start. My heart sank into my boots at the thought of a raw, burning throat for at least 4 weeks and not able to eat anything but pureed food. There was also the future problem of maybe not being able to swallow due to the radiation narrowing the oesophagus, and having to undergo yet another operation for it to be rectified.

The oncologist recommended having a CT scan of the head, neck, chest and abdomen before going on holiday, and for treatment to commence soon after returning from the US. I mentioned to Phil that once I was on the cruise ship I would not want to come home; what with poor Mum to worry about and my own upcoming painful treatment, I might even think about chucking myself off the side of the boat on the last day.

Wednesday 15th February saw me sitting in the Nuffield hospital again at Cambridge waiting for a CT scan. First I had to drink almost a jugful of water with a tasteless contrast added, and I had an hour to do it in. Unfortunately I was awash with liquid at the end of it and could not manage to drink the full jug. Another type of contrast was added by IV injection halfway through the scan, causing a hot flush and my heart to palpitate alarmingly. My oncologist emailed me the results of the scan just before we left for Heathrow, and the treatment side-effects, which were even more alarming:

'Glenda has had a recent ultrasound, which unfortunately has shown a small recurrence on the right side of the thyroid bed measuring 12 x 7mm.

I explained to Glenda that we had discussed the potential options in our recent thyroid MDT which could include the consideration of further surgery, although this would be potentially difficult because of the problems with her prior vocal cord palsy. The alternative, as we have discussed previously, would be to consider her for localised radiotherapy to the neck.

On balance today we have opted to go for radiotherapy treatment. Prior to starting this I will repeat thyroglobulin with antibody measurement to see if this has increased, and will also arrange a CT staging scan to make sure there is no evidence of disease elsewhere. If the CT staging scan is clear, then we will proceed to radiotherapy to a dose of 60 Gy in 30 fractions delivered over 6 weeks. I have explained this to Glenda today, and explained that in the short term the side effects that may occur include soreness of the skin, difficulty and painful swallowing, and the need for strong analgesia. She knows that she will need an altered diet, and may lose some hair on the posterior of her neck. This should re-grow. She knows that swallowing may become more difficult and that she will have regular input from dietitians and speech and language therapists. In the long term the risks associated with this treatment are small. We will keep her spinal cord and brain stem within safe tolerance. There can be risk of oesophageal strictures in the future.'

Oh, deepest joy!

We set off for Heathrow on 18th February for an overnight stay. I tried to put all thoughts of my upcoming treatment out of my head and enjoy the cruise. I asked Lee and Matthew to keep me updated regarding Mum; I felt terribly guilty for leaving her in a nursing home, but she told me to go off and enjoy myself.

We boarded a Virgin Atlantic plane bound for Miami on 19th February, and arrived to blazing sunshine about 8 hours later. There was another overnight stay in a Miami hotel, and then we were transferred to our cruise ship the next day. We had a wonderful holiday, taking in Grand Cayman, swimming with dolphins in Costa Maya, visiting Cozumel, and of course sailing up the Mississippi river and arriving in New Orleans just in time for the Mardi Gras celebrations. Our sons told me that Mum was doing okay in her new nursing home, and I started to relax and enjoy myself.

Only one cloud spoiled the whole cruising experience as waited in the rain on the dock at Georgetown, Grand Cayman, on 22nd February for the last tender to take us back to our cruise ship. The skies were black, and I hoped we would get back to the safety of the ship, which had been anchored in deeper waters, before the storm really began. The excursion supervisor looked up and assured us it would only be one of those squally showers that can afflict Georgetown in February, and we had no doubt that the sun would soon return from behind the clouds.

A howling wind whipped frothy waves up over our sandals as we waited. I looked at my watch; the ship would be sailing at 4pm, and the last tender was due to leave at 3.30. It was already 3.20. A few of us hardy souls had taken a longer than average trolley ride around the capital, braving the inclement weather and singing to the driver while he had unrolled plastic sheeting down the sides of the trolley in a futile attempt to keep us dry.

By 3.45 and with no sign of the rain abating, we boarded a bobbing tender. The ship had a tight schedule, and tardy guests missing the deadline had to make their own way to the next port of call, which was hundreds of miles away. A local company had provided the means of transporting three thousand cruise passengers from ship to shore and back again, and so the cruise ship's own orange tenders (doubling as lifeboats) had not been launched that day.

As the tender rocked and rolled in the howling wind, I was glad I hadn't eaten anything since breakfast. Passengers cheered as wave after wave splashed up over them, but all I wanted to do was get back to the relative stability of the huge ship. The up and down motion of a small boat had never been a favourite of mine. I closed my eyes and wished the moments away.

I felt the height of the waves increase. Phil informed me with some concern that they looked to be at least ten feet high. I didn't want to open my eyes. I could hear passengers still cheering. Phil laughed and told me we had reached the ship, and that passengers were performing Mexican waves as the boat was tossed about. I opened my eyes and saw the ship's crew standing in the gangway on deck 2 waiting to receive us. Our little boat bashed against the sides of the ship, the engine strained, and it was obvious to all and sundry that we could not dock.

As the boat struggled to stay upright in the wind and waves, the crew of the tender began to hand us out life jackets. A long pole was retrieved from its moorings above, and placed on the floor. Suddenly the passengers ceased to cheer, and all that could be heard over the noise of the engine was one woman vomiting into a plastic bag.

My heart was racing with a burst of adrenaline as I struggled to don my life jacket. I heard Phil say that he could swim better and keep me afloat without the hindrance of a great orange thing around his neck, and he refused to wear one. Other passengers old, infirm, or hugely overweight also did not bother to put on theirs. I was terrified that our boys would lose both parents at the same time, and wanted the best chance of survival. I asked a crew member to help me fasten the lifejacket straps properly. He told me he was used to rough seas, and not to worry.

Several ship's officers were looking at us with concern from the gangway, and smug cruisers regarded us as entertainment and watched our plight from the safety of their balconies on the upper decks. Officers radioed to the boat's captain to return us to the port so that we could board a larger tender. My heart sank as we moved away from virtual rescue and back into the open sea again.

The vomiting lady excelled herself all the way back to port, where a larger tender had appeared. Soaking wet, terrified, and clutching my damp rucksack, I reluctantly boarded the vessel with Phil, who cuddled me all the way back to the cruise ship with two cold, wet arms.

The rain stopped as suddenly as it had begun, the sun came out, and we were at last able to be transferred safely back to the cruise ship. As I walked through the security scanner, I was dismayed to be greeted with a cup of steaming hot milky chocolate. I am dairy intolerant!

***

The rest of the holiday went without a hitch, and of course the Mardi Gras celebrations were awesome. We strolled down Bourbon Street and caught beads thrown from balconies. We also signed up for tours that took in the iconic Lafayette cemetery number 1, and also an old Louisiana plantation, Houmas House.

CHAPTER 52 – DEATH OF MY MOTHER

It was as though Mum was waiting for us to return. We had only been back for one day when I received the 3am phone call that we were dreading. Mum was slipping away. She died hours later on Sunday March 5th 2017. I was glad that we were able to visit her before she died. She was not fully conscious and was receiving morphine through a syringe driver, but she could squeeze my hand if I asked her to. I informed the funeral directors that Mum's pre-existing plan would now need to be put into action, and the funeral was arranged for March 30th 2017 at 10.30am.

I had been taking care of Mum's finances and in fact doing quite a lot for her for the last two years of her life. I knew that Mum had put some money by for me, and I knew what I was going to do with it. I had discussed with Mum buying a holiday home on our beloved Isle of Wight, and Mum had been all for it. Therefore taking my near brush with death into account on the tender, and in case my upcoming treatment might not ultimately be effective, I decided that there was no time like the present to seize the day. I got in touch with the holiday homes' sales assistant Phil and I had seen the previous autumn, and we put a deposit down on a a lovely static caravan near St. Helens.

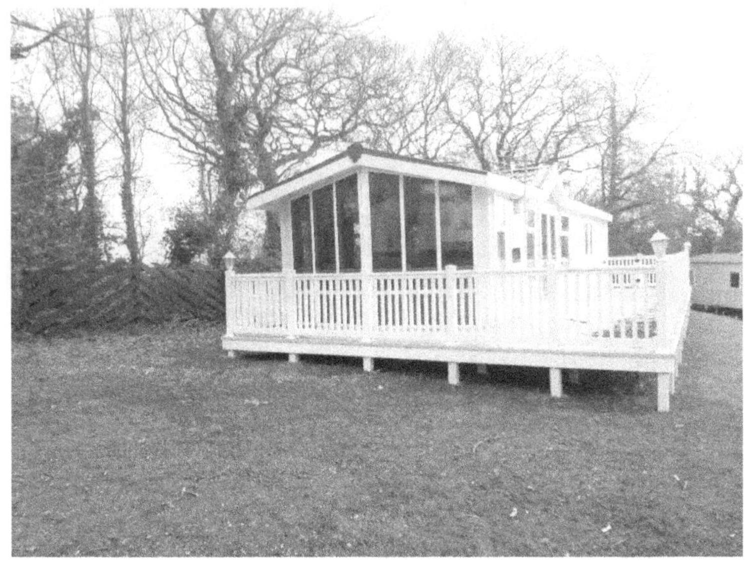

On top of funeral arranging and sorting out Mum's possessions, I had to begin attending Addenbrooke's hospital for the commencement of my treatment. I also had to attend the Spire Lea hospital for a dental assessment, as the radiation could involve my lower jaw. I dreaded losing my teeth; this year of our Lord 2017 was definitely not my year! At the Spire Lea I had to have an x-ray of my jaws and teeth (I wondered how much radiation my body could take), but the facial surgeon could not see any problems. Before he had even started his investigations he marked me out as a tooth grinder (because my teeth were 'flat') and a non-smoker (because I had no vertical lines above my top lip). How clever! He prescribed me some high fluoride toothpaste and a high fluoride mouthwash, Endekay, to offset necrosis of the jaw and tooth loss due to the radiation, which I would have to take twice a day for life. Joy.

On 13th March I presented at the Radiotherapy Department in Oncology, where I was informed that a mask was to be made for me right there and then. I had to take off my top clothes and earrings, and lie on the bed of the tomography machine. Something like a hot blanket with holes in was put over my face and the top half of my chest (I kept my eyes shut), and this was clamped down to the tomography bed, rendering me immobile. The heat left the mask-blanket, and it hardened around my face. A most unpleasant experience, and I knew I had to wear the damn thing every time I was laid under the machine until the end of my treatment date on 10th May. The mask would again be clamped to the tomography bed each time, and I would have to endure the whole process as best I could for the 20 or so minutes while blasts of radiation hopefully killed off my tumour(s).

The radiotherapy assistant suggested bringing in a CD to listen to and to concentrate on. This made sense to me. I ordered an audio book and bought a cheap portable CD player, as I thought listening to a story would involve more concentration than listening to music, and therefore it might be easier to take my mind away from what was happening.

I managed to persuade the receptionists to book me evening appointments, so that Phil could drive me if I was not feeling well. In this way he would be able to hold down his job without causing too many problems for his customers and employers.

Just before the actual treatment started I had appointments with a dietitian, a skin care nurse, and a speech and language therapist. The dietitian recommended eating a high carb diet to keep the calories up, and the skin care nurse told me to use E45 cream on my neck and keep it regularly moisturised. The speech and language therapist measured how far I could open my mouth (the opening is reduced in the first place because of the meniscectomy of the left jaw I had undergone back in 2006), and told me that my irradiated throat might cause food to 'go down the wrong way', and that I should be careful when eating and might also need to change my diet to a puree one for the last few weeks of treatment.

Even deeper joy. My nights prior to the first treatment were restless. I would wake up around 2am remembering the feel of the mask over my face and the entrapment, and dread the thought of having to wear it almost every day for 6 weeks.

The first day of the treatment dawned on Monday March 27th. I was so nervous when Phil was driving me there that I hardly said a word. When we arrived at the Radiotherapy Department there was a little bit of a heartsink moment; only one tomography machine was working, and there was a backup of patients. The waiting room was overflowing, and we were told to come back in an hour. We walked around, found a café, and I read my Kindle and Phil bought a Sudoku book. By the time I was called for treatment over 2 hours had passed since my appointment time, and I was more angry than nervous when the put the mask over my face and adjusted it so that it wasn't too tight. The scanner was noisy, and I wasn't able to hear my audio book. I decided to bring a music CD the following evening. We arrived home at 10pm!

After four lots of radiotherapy I was getting used to the mask, but my lower gum was already red and sore, and I could no longer tolerate hot drinks. I hoped to God I wasn't going to lose my teeth after 6 weeks of it. The worst day of 2017 was Thursday 30th March, as Mum's funeral was in the morning, and I had a treatment in the evening. My granddaughter Caitlin had a lovely idea of doing a balloon release in the garden after the funeral though, which went off very well. It was a sunny, cloudless day, very unusual for late March, and the 20 helium-filled balloons were soon flying around the stratosphere. I hope that Mum saw them.

CHAPTER 53 – MORE RADIATION AND AFTER -EFFECTS

We escaped to the Isle of Wight on the weekend after my first treatment to pay the outstanding balance on our holiday home and finalise the paperwork. We had been talking about doing this for years, and now with my inheritance from Mum and no firm guarantee that the treatment would cure the cancer, I decided there was no time like the present. Phil drove and I slept all the way there and all the way back, but it was lovely to be on the Island we love and to finally take possession of a beautiful home that we could come and go from as we wished. I hoped I would be well enough to visit the Island again a fortnight later at Easter.

After 5 days of being irradiated the mouth sores started to appear. They would flare up as soon as I got up off the tomography machine, and would calm down again the following day, only to reappear again in force with another treatment. I started to use frequent salt mouthwashes and made sure I used Endekay twice a day. My oncologist prescribed Difflam mouthwash and Nystatin, which seemed to help. I also took my food blender down from a high shelf, gave it a good wash, and began to juice raw organic vegetables. The taste was less than pleasant, but I wanted to put some goodness into my body to try and counteract the radiation.

After 10 days of radiotherapy my reflux had worsened and the expected sore throat appeared. I was prescribed Omeprazole liquid to take at night, as all my usual strategies to counteract reflux had failed except sitting upright and staying awake! I also had to step up the All Bran at breakfast time to aid the poor old bowels, which were struggling somewhat with having to take the maximum allowed dose of anti-emetics. It also started taking me ages to eat anything, as I had to chew on a very small amount of food and swallow it with a sip of water.

On 9th April we took Mum's ashes down to her mother Harriet's grave in East London. Lee, Matt, Anna and their two boys accompanied us. Phil dug a large hole in the middle of the grave for the casket, and then covered it over with earth and stones so that nobody could have even guessed we'd been there. We tidied up the grave and re-painted the frame. I'm sure Mum would have approved of her final resting place. She had always hated Suffolk, and often pined for the East London of her youth.

By 12th April my throat was very sore indeed, and all I could taste was salt. Normal toothpaste made my mouth feel as though it was burning. Another eye infection appeared in my right eye. I began to wonder how on earth I could withstand another 17 treatments. On the next day the hair at the back of my head began to fall out and I felt nauseous. A visit to the oncologist for a review saw me coming away with a bagful of medications to manage the side effects; Codeine, Ondansetron, Cyclizine, Paracetamol, Lactulose, Senna, and more Omeprazole. She told me that people withstood the whole course of treatments because they were medically optimised for the side-effects, whereas I had not been. She also let slip that she was due to have an operation to remove part of her thyroid gland! I didn't like to ask if it was cancerous, and I wondered if it had been damaged by too many visits to her patients whilst they were undergoing radioactive iodine treatment.

By the end of 12 treatments on 21st April everything tasted of salt, my mouth was as dry as the desert, and without extensive anti-emetics I felt as though I constantly wanted to either retch or throw up. The skin on my neck was red raw, and I wanted to sleep all day. Constipation was a problem unless I quadrupled the dose of laxatives. I saw a new doctor for my review on that Friday, who prescribed an artificial saliva gel, more anti-emetics, and a nebuliser for increased secretions. I was desperate for it all to end, and it really was a case of mind over matter to be immobilised in the tomography machine when any minute I felt that I might vomit.

Strangely enough by the start of the 5th week of treatment the sore throat had eased somewhat, and I didn't feel the need to take paracetamol tablets until the following week. However, constipation and nausea were problematic, and I had lost over half a stone in weight and felt permanently tired. By the 6th week the skin on the front of my neck was not only red raw and sore, it was peeling and oozing as well. One of the Addenbrooke's doctors prescribed Flamazine, a silver sulphadiazine cream given to patients suffering from burns, because of course my neck was in the same state as anybody who'd had damage from a burn, no matter how they had received it. Flamazine is excellent, and the skin healed fairly quickly, although not on the inside of my throat.

After the penultimate treatment some enamel broke off one of my teeth while I was chewing a sausage roll. I wondered if this was due to an irradiated lower jaw or the fact that I couldn't wear my mouth guard at night (due to retching) and so was constantly grinding my teeth when I was asleep. I knew my dentist would not want to work on this particular tooth, which he had previously temporarily filled and stated that any further treatment would be root canal work. I therefore made an appointment to see the oral surgeon I had visited before my radiotherapy treatment commenced. A quick visit to the dentist reassured me that nothing was dreadfully amiss and that I did not need the attention of an oral surgeon. The dentist repaired my tooth there and then.

The last day of radiotherapy treatment was May 10th 2017. By then I had lost nearly one stone in weight, and had a nasty sore throat and reduced ability to swallow, and hardly any appetite as well as a red raw, virtually immobile neck (one of the radiographers admitted that 'you neck guys get it the worst'). Quite a lot of my hair had fallen out at the back of my neck, and all food tasted of salt. I was the last patient to be seen in the evening, and when I came out of the treatment room there was nobody else around. I felt like doing a little dance to celebrate, but was too tired. The radiographer followed me out and asked if I'd like to keep my mask/shell. My answer was very firmly in the negative!

After 2 weeks I had ditched all the tablets except the Omeprazole and didn't feel sick anymore, but still none of the food I ate tasted like it should. My throat was still sore, although not as much, and I couldn't swallow without sipping water at the same time as lumps of food. I could not put on any weight, and the scales stayed stubbornly at 9 stones. However, I could now wear a small mouth guard to protect my teeth at night, but didn't feel ready to tackle the bigger one I had previously worn.

After 4 weeks I still weighed 9 stones, but at least my weight was stable. My throat was still faintly sore, my mouth was dry and the swallowing still not back to normal, but my voice had recovered. There was no sign of hair re-growth at the back of my head. My taste buds had been massacred; even water tasted strange, and I had to drink water from our filter instead. I still felt as though I wanted to retch all the time. However, I could lie down and sleep on my side again at night, and didn't need to doze so much during the day.

Had the treatment worked? I had no idea, as I now had to wait about three months for everything to heal and settle back into place before I could have a scan. I decided to eat as much good food as I could, and enjoy the summer. To have something to look forward to I booked more visits to our holiday home on the Isle of Wight for the end of May bank holiday, for the owners' summer ball at the end of June, for another few days with our granddaughters at the end of July, for 3 days at the end of August, and for a week with Phil's sister and her husband at the beginning of September. I was also buoyed and encouraged by finding my first five star review for 'Living With Thyroid Cancer' on Amazon:

"This book was really informative re thyroid cancer. I have this condition and presently going for my 2nd RAI treatment. I read the book that Glenda wrote for beginners too. This is the 2nd time that I have picked this book up; the 1st time prior to my two ops, and again before treatment. It gives me informed facts plus the unselfish sharing of herself…experiences, feelings, thoughts etc, and allows valuable identification of the thyroid journey. Many thanks."

I also decided to go back to work part-time as a bank secretary to cover holidays and sickness, and went to see my old manager and Occupational Health to get the ball rolling at the beginning of July. I wanted to be able to contribute to the running of our holiday home, which as far as I could tell, was going to cost us in the region of about £600 per month. The fees for 2017 were all included in the original price, and so come October we would need to set up a direct debit with the park's finance department and start paying for the privilege of owning a home on such a beautiful part of the Island.

I was given the all-clear to start work again. My manager then sent me dates for training on the new hospital system that had been installed while I had been away. I was a medical secretary again, albeit a 'bank' one.

CHAPTER 54 - LYMPHOEDEMA

On July 7th I had a follow up with my oncologist at the Nuffield Hospital, Cambridge. Two months since the treatment ended and my mouth was still as dry as the desert (I was having to eat and sip water at the same time). However, I had stopped the Omeprazole due to muscle aches, and my taste buds were beginning to recover, especially the sweet tastes. The consultant said it could be two more years before my salivary glands recovered, if they ever did, as they had taken a 'pasting' with previous radioiodine treatments. She told me my hair would start to re-grow about three months after the treatment (it was still sparse at the back of my head). My right eye still watered intermittently.

I had some bloods taken for thyroxine levels, as I had stayed at 9 stone in weight and was concerned that I was on too much medication. I was told that I would be sent an appointment the following month for an ultrasound to check whether I was once again in remission, as the radiation was still working in my body and would be for 3 months following the last appointment on 10th May.

I dreaded this scan taking place on 29th August. It was becoming patently obvious to me that all but one of my treatment options had been used up, never to be repeated. I could have no more surgery (due to internal scarring) or radiotherapy (any more would be dangerous). The only treatment left would be the sorafenib tablets, the side-effects of which might cause me to feel permanently unwell.

While the sun shone during July I buried my head in the sand and tried not to think about it.

The results of my blood test came back, and as far as my oncologist was concerned, I was on the correct dose of thyroxine. She told me to stay on 100mcg four times per week and 125mcg three times per week until I saw her again on 17th November, when repeat bloods would be taken.

Another symptom manifested itself 3 months following the last radiotherapy treatment. Every morning my neck would be swollen, particularly under the chin, making swallowing difficult. After I had been upright and moving about for an hour or so, the swelling would decrease and I could carefully eat my breakfast. I sent an email to my oncologist, who told me that lymphoedema was a common occurrence after treatment, and to sleep propped up and to massage the neck in an outwards direction each morning. Normal lymph channels had been damaged through surgery and radiation, and the fluid was having trouble draining. There was even a name for the under-chin swelling, 'Dewlap Lymphoedema'. When I emailed back to ask if the swelling decreased with time, she did not reply! What she did do was to refer me to the lymphoedema specialist nurses, who would be able to find new drainage channels for my lymph fluid. Apparently it can be done through massage I think.

***

Yet again my heart was pounding as I lay on the couch for an ultrasound scan at the end of August 2017. As usual the doctor did not say much as he applied the gel and ran the probe over my neck. However, to my utter surprise and delight he eventually told me after a few minutes of me living in dread that the scan was clear! All the pain and discomfort had been worth it – I was now cancer-free again.

I do not know how long I will be free of papillary thyroid cancer.

It could be for the rest of my life, or the cancer may come back. I have no idea. What I do know is that I'm going to enjoy every day I have left, accept the side-effects of radiation, and enjoy my lovely family, my holiday home, my job, and my LIFE!!

THE LEGACY OF THYROID CANCER

ALTERED SENSATION

I've had extensive treatment to the neck area to rid me of my cancer. Unfortunately this has caused my neck to feel quite differently these days. Three surgeries and 30 sessions of external beam radiotherapy have caused much internal scarring and lymphoedema. My neck isn't as supple as it used to be as regards turning, and the accumulation of fluid around my neck and upper chest often gives me the sensation that I'm carrying a bucket of water around in that area.

The two neck dissection surgeries also affected the shoulders, which sometimes feel stiff. I do my upper body exercises religiously every morning to keep things moving. The shoulder joints creak and groan, but there's no way I'm going to have another painful cortisone injection into my shoulder joint ever again!

ALTERED TASTE

When I first underwent external beam radiotherapy (EBR), all foods except bacon and crisps tasted of salt. Therefore I tended to like to eat bacon and crisps (neither of which I usually eat as I do not like salty food) because they tasted as they should.

A year on from EBR and my taste buds have recovered. However, there are some foods I like to eat now that I didn't before, and vice versa. I cannot tolerate bananas nor porridge now, two of my favourite staples, but crave oranges instead. Oranges used to make me feel nauseous, but now they don't – how weird is that? Also I find that alcohol burns my throat, so I don't drink it anymore.

ANXIETY

Will the cancer return or won't it? I expect every person who has ever suffered with cancer has worried about this at some point or another, usually every time they experience a pain somewhere or have a persistent cough for example.

My cancer has returned three times, but this time I hope it has gone for good. Every time it returned when I least expected it and when I had become quite blasé about the whole experience. As long as you have regular check-ups and scans, and don't ignore any bodily changes, then any recurrence will have a chance of being caught early.

I often think to myself that it's useless to keep on worrying about whether or not the cancer will return, as all the worrying in the world will not stop it coming back. In fact the worrying could cause extra stress anyway, which is not good for us. However, it is difficult not to think about recurrence – I know, as I've been there myself, but after a few clear scans the worrying does get a little bit less.

DRY EYES

Eye problems started quite early on in my treatment, about 2 years after the first doses of radioactive iodine back in 2006. I first experienced watery eyes every time I stepped outside in the cold air, which was annoying. Next came sore eyes and frequent bouts of conjunctivitis in both eyes, which was miserable and distressing. I also awoke with terribly dry eyes at night, which were painful to move.

Radiation narrows the nasolacrimal ducts, and tears cannot drain away properly down the back of the nose. This was confirmed by syringing my tear ducts, where saline gushed down my cheeks instead of down the back of my throat.

I had two operations; an external dacryocystorhinostomy (DCR) in the left eye where I ended up with a small scar on my nose, and a year later an internal DCR for the right eye. The internal DCR never worked as well, and my right eye still waters and becomes inflamed from time to time. However, the nasolacrimal duct is open, and there's not much more the surgeon can do for me.

I use Hylo Forte drops for the dry eyes, and have Chloramphenicol ointment on repeat prescription so that I can use it straight away when an attack of conjunctivitis arrives. Other than these I frequently splash cold water on my eyes, which helps too.

DRY MOUTH

Even after 4 doses of radioactive iodine I still didn't have a dry mouth. However, a few years' later after 30 sessions of external beam radiotherapy my poor old salivary glands took a pasting. I now have a permanently dry mouth and have to sip water very frequently. I also have to sip water when eating solid food, as otherwise I cannot swallow it unless it has gravy or some sort of sauce.

There are moisturising mouth sprays available. I've tried a few but didn't get on with them. However, 'Oralieve' doesn't seem to be too bad, and it saves on the need to constantly drink. It's handy if I'm out somewhere though, but at home I prefer to sip water.

Having next to no saliva also means that my teeth are more prone to decay. I have to use 'Endekay' mouth wash twice a day, and brush my teeth twice a day with 'Duraphat' toothpaste, which is high in fluoride. I clean my teeth after each meal, and even take a toothbrush and toothpaste out with me. It's a bit of a pain at work as there is only one toilet and I'm in there ages after lunch cleaning my teeth, but it has to be done. My gnashers haven't fallen out yet, and I'm taking great care to make sure they don't.

Another disadvantage (or maybe it is an advantage now) I've found through having a dry mouth is that I cannot suck on any boiled sweets otherwise I will retch. Dry heaving seems to accompany a dry mouth, at least it does with me. I've found out that as well as the dry mouth, it's all to do with increased sensitivity of the throat after radiation, which I will write about later in the book.

HEAT ISSUES / LOW TSH

My oncologist likes to keep me slightly over-medicated on thyroxine to keep the TSH suppressed (under 0.1), but hopefully this is not enough to cause brittle bones or heart disease. However, it does make me intolerant to heat.

When I first had my thyroidectomy I was started off on 200mcg of thyroxine. Within a short time my glasses were steaming up on the inside and my heart was pounding as though I'd just run a marathon! Not good.

Nowadays it's taken a bit of tweaking, but I generally feel well on 100mcg 5 days per week, 125mcg 2 days per week, and with an extra 25mcg every other week.

If I go anywhere where the temperature is above 20 degrees Celsius I begin to feel too hot. Family and friends know that a wall of heat is **not** going to greet them when I open my front door, and some of them even put on an extra jumper if they visit (my mother, bless her, used to leave her coat on). Fortunately my husband shares the same heat issues as I do.

I have been in some people's houses where I have ended up standing outside in the garden to cool off. These heat issues are never – ending, and whoop-de-do-dah for the last 8 years I've had the double whammy of menopausal hot flushes as well, which combine sweatily with my thyroxine over-medication to ensure that I hardly ever need to wear a coat!

The menopausal flushes are grinding to a halt these days, and I only tend to have them first thing in the mornings. However, I am still unaccountably hot most of the time.

HOARSE VOICE

You may be lucky and get away with it, but I wasn't. My hoarse voice started straight after my thyroidectomy back in June 2015. I soon found out why – one of my vocal cords had been paralysed during the operation. All that came out was a whisper for 6 whole months. My sons were in seventh heaven because I couldn't yell at them…

But even this had a silver lining. With not much of a voice I had to be re-deployed at work as I couldn't speak to patients or their relatives and couldn't answer the phone. I was promoted from a grade 2 ward clerk to a grade 3 medical secretary. Grade 3s do not have to answer the phone and can just type clinic letters. This was great for me, and a year after the operation I was promoted to a grade 4 medical secretary when my voice had returned from wherever it had been taking its holiday.

Unfortunately though my left vocal cord never recovered and is still paralysed today, giving me a slightly reduced airway and a croaky voice. My voice has been made worse over the years by successive radiotherapy treatments – the last one consisting of 30 external beam radiotherapy sessions that burnt the inside of my throat and almost killed my voice completely.

A year on, and the voice is rallying round a little bit. I've actually got a range of 5 notes that I can sing! Woop-de-do-dah. I sound like a constipated corncrake when I warble to my heart's content in the bath, but I suppose it's better than having no voice at all.

Yes I've been to a few speech therapists, blown copious bubbles through straws and have been mindful to try and clear my throat instead of coughing, which apparently my right vocal cord prefers. Sorry to disappoint it, but sometimes a good old cough just has to be done.

Also, having radiotherapy can cause increased phlegm at the back of the throat, which also affects the quality of the voice. I've suffered with increased phlegm ever since my first radioiodine treatment, and unfortunately it takes years to decrease.

INCREASED SENSITIVITY OF THE THROAT

I found out in the most unpleasant way how much more sensitive any bodily tissue is that has been subject to external beam radiotherapy. I was prescribed Carbamazepine by a neurologist for glossopharyngeal neuralgia which I've had since I was a teenager. However, it has been made worse by the radiotherapy.

I had a strange inkling that I'd better be careful taking any new drug that my body was not used to, so I only took half a tablet before bedtime. Six hours' later I woke up with a pounding heart, which is a sign I recognise when my body doesn't like something. Unfortunately soon after this I felt my throat begin to close up. I couldn't talk, and it was becoming rather difficult to breathe. I've never had this before, and tried not to panic.

I woke Phil up, and he drove me straight to Accident & Emergency without waiting for an ambulance. They injected me with IV steroids and anti-histamines straight away. Within about half an hour the swelling in my throat began to subside, and they kept me in a quiet room for a few hours.

This episode has made me very mindful of taking any new prescription medication.

I have also noticed my throat is more sensitive to certain types of fruit (grapes for example) and also alcohol. I don't drink alcohol at all these days, and am trying not to have to make a repeat visit to A&E!

Funnily enough, after taking just one Carbamazepine tablet, my glossopharyngeal neuralgia never returned!

LYMPHOEDEMA OF THE NECK

I did not come across this unwelcome addition to my symptoms until about 3 months after I had undergone 30 sessions of external beam radiotherapy (EBR). One morning I woke up and my neck felt strangely heavy and peculiar, and what was more alarming, I could not swallow a thing (*wtf?* Another *'oma'* in my throat?)

After about an hour of being upright and walking about I could swallow again and my neck did not feel so heavy and strange, but I had no idea what had caused this to happen. Over the next few mornings it happened again, and I re-read the advice and guidance leaflet that had been given to me at the start of my EBR which was still sitting where I'd left it when I'd first brought it home from hospital. Low and behold, under the heading of 'Lymphoedema', I found symptoms similar to mine.

After reading more about it on Google, I realised with dismay that I now had a lifelong condition which I would have to learn to manage. When I went back to Addenbrooke's Hospital for a check-up I mentioned the collection of fluid around my neck, and the Speech & Language Department put me in touch with a lymphoedema nurse nearer to my home.

The lymphoedema nurse was a specialist in head and neck lymphoedema. She measured my neck and suggested a couple of things to help me, which I have described below:

A MASSAGE ROLLER:

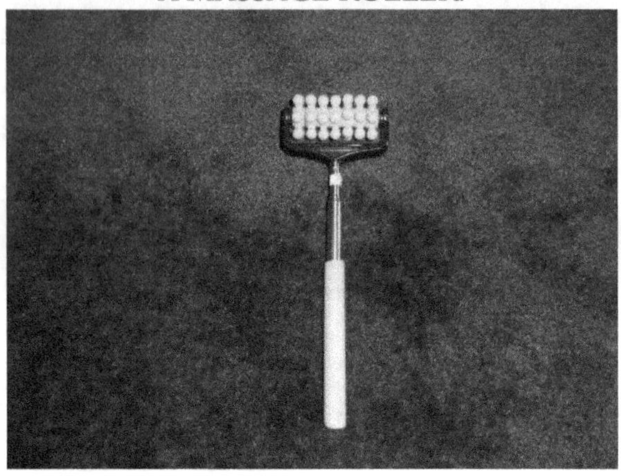

Very inexpensive, the roller is a must-have little device which helps shift unwanted fluid from around the neck, or in fact anywhere else in the body I would imagine. Mine cost around £3.50.

After a couple of months my neck was measured again, and the measurements were less than at the start. I use the roller every day, and will do ad infinitum!

Another device to use is this Velcro collar, which to me looks just like a sanitary towel, but hey ho, thank goodness I've no need for those anymore:

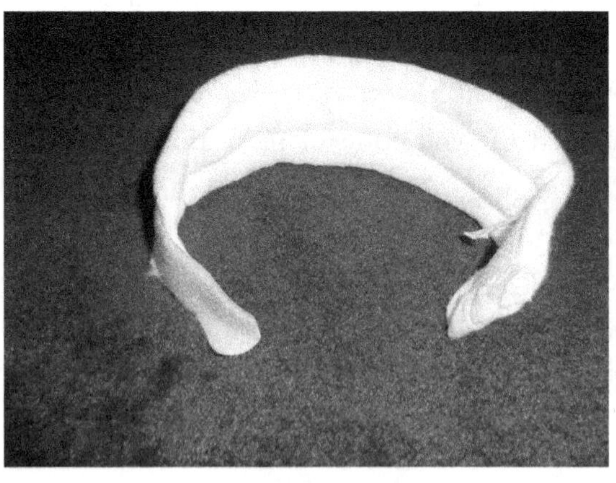

Also the trick is to sleep on your back as upright as you can manage, with your head tilted back (if you let it loll forwards the fluid will collect under the chin). If you wake in the night, give your neck a bit of a rogering with the roller.

So yeah, it sucks that you can't lay down in your bed at night, but you soon get used to sleeping half propped up. And because you're half upright, your neck doesn't fill up with fluid as much as when you're laying down and you get to drink your cup of whatever first thing in the morning and it actually goes down your throat!

NECK DISSECTIONS:

Two years after the thyroidectomy I found out the cancer had spread to the lymph nodes on the left side of my neck. In 2007 I underwent a left radical neck dissection, a 6 hour operation where the surgeon removed suspicious-looking neck tissue. He found many cancerous lymph nodes, but afterwards the cancer never came back on that side. It took many months to recover from such a major operation (after the op I had a long scar from my ear down to the middle of my neck and 110 metal staples in the side of my neck), and of course there was permanent altered sensation and numbness.

Seven years' later when I'd been in remission for seven years, the cancer came back on the right side and I had to undergo a further right sided radical neck dissection. I now have a scar running from ear to ear, but it has faded with time and I don't really think about it much now.

NECK STIFFNESS

If I did not carry out my morning stretching exercises, then my neck stiffness would become worse. My neck does feel rather strange in the mornings when I get out of bed, but following a half an hour of stretching out my lower back and neck muscles, this usually makes me feel something akin to normal again.

After the first neck dissection operation, my surgeon was quick to point out that if I did not get my neck moving, then it would stiffen up completely. I cannot stress this point enough, as he was definitely correct.

To offset neck lymphoedema I have to sleep in one position only; virtually sitting upright with my head tilted back on 6 pillows – not conducive to neck flexibility! For 58 years I slept on my side using two pillows, but no more… it's no use bemoaning the fact that I cannot sleep how I want to. I have to get used to the 'new normal'. I have had thyroid cancer, and it's a life-changing experience.

RECURRENCE OF THYROID CANCER

Of course once you have had cancer and have been in remission for some time, the worry is that it will return. After the first recurrence I was in remission for 7 years and thought I'd got rid of thyroid cancer for good, but no, back it came again and I had to deal with it. The only option I had left after 4 doses of radioactive iodine, one thyroidectomy and 2 neck dissections was External Beam Radiotherapy (EBR) – 30 doses. I would have to lie under a tomography machine for 20 minutes every working day for 6 weeks, with my face encased in a mask which had to be clamped to the scan table to ensure that I stayed immobile so the radiation could then be directed to where it was supposed to go.

To start with I had an appointment at Addenbrooke's Hospital where they made the mask that I would have to wear for all 30 sessions. The radiographers laid hot, wet material over my face, neck, and the upper part of my chest, all the while telling me to breathe normally. The material hardened within a short time to fit the contours of my face, and I could see through it. Then I had appointments with Speech & Language and Dietetics departments to learn the side-effects of the treatment that I might experience.

I think I experienced most of them; feeling sick, painful swallowing, changes in taste, dry lips and mouth, inflamed, red skin, constipation, and a worsening of my reflux (a good thing a year later about not being able to lie down at night is that the reflux problem disappears!). I was dosed up on so much medication that I nicknamed Phil 'The Pharmacy King', as whenever I attended follow up appointments he had to queue for ages at Addenbrooke's pharmacy to collect my list of tablets to help me cope with the treatment. Here's my little list and their effects, but after the treatment had ended I was able to come off all of them within a short space of time.

- Omeprazole: Helps with reflux.
- Soluble Paracetamol: Helps with painful swallowing.
- Senna: Laxative. The normal dose has to be quadrupled to ease constipation.
- Lactulose: Another laxative.
- Flamizine: Anti-burn cream to apply to neck skin.
- Domperidone: Anti-emetic.
- Ondansetron: A stronger anti-emetic that causes bad constipation.
- Codeine: Painkiller.

Yes it's a bloody awful scenario when the cancer returns and you wonder whether you're going to survive. I certainly thought my time was up, but hey, after the EBR I have had a year so far without any recurrence.

RETCHING

Yet another miserable condition caused by the external beam radiotherapy sessions. The body's tissues, especially inside the mouth and throat, become permanently more sensitive. This has caused me to often feel like retching. To avoid embarrassing myself in public I always carry a bottle of water with me, and drink this to offset the urge to retch.

Another problem is that I cannot tolerate any dental work at the back of my mouth, and now have to undergo an anaesthetic for fillings to my back teeth. I can just about tolerate work on the front teeth, but oh, the back teeth are a whole new ball game. I am always cleaning my teeth to avoid tooth decay!

SHOULDER STIFFNESS

As soon as I had the first neck dissection operation on the left side back in 2007 I experienced a sore shoulder. After a couple of years this shoulder was as stiff as a board, and I could hardly raise my arm. I had to undergo a terribly painful cortisone injection into my shoulder joint to ease the pain and stiffness. After another neck dissection on the right side I was determined not to acquire a stiff right shoulder. Every morning I complete my routine shoulder, neck and back exercises based on ones from the Pilates class I attended for about 18 months.

So far the right shoulder hasn't stiffened up, although the left side often feels sore and stiff sometimes. I still cannot bend my left arm back as far as the right arm.

SLEEPING ISSUES

Sleeping was fine until I 'acquired' lymphoedema of the neck. Now I have to sleep virtually sitting up with my head tilted backwards, otherwise I would wake up with a swollen neck and be unable to swallow. I've got used to it now after a year, and funnily enough this new sleeping position plus a memory foam mattress ensures that I never wake up with low backache like I used to when I slept lower down on my side.

SWOLLEN SALIVARY GLANDS

These were mostly a problem after the first dose of radioactive iodine back in 2006. I could feel the salivary glands swelling as I chewed, and tried to ensure I ate soft moist foods to help them out. They briefly swelled up again after the external beam radiotherapy, which more or less finished them off. Now I have to sip water with food in order to swallow it, because I have almost no saliva at all.

THYROXINE ISSUES

I've been lucky in this department, as apart from when the doctors first tried me with Levothyroxine and put me on too high a dose (my glasses steamed up on the inside and my heart was pounding as though I'd run a marathon!) my body has taken to it quite well. I'm on rather a bespoke dose though, in order to keep the thyroxine stimulating hormone suppressed and to offset any heart palpitations and heat issues.

I have to take 100mcg 5 times a week, 125mcg twice a week, and an extra 25mcg every other week. It's a good thing I don't suffer with Alzheimer's disease! The optimum thyroxine dose depends on your weight and how active you are. If you take thyroxine and suddenly gain or lose weight, you may find you are either hypo or hyperthyroid. It's best to keep your weight stable and not go climbing mountains or running 5 marathons in a row.

***

So there you have it. I am alive and currently cancer-free, but you can see by reading this that anybody who says thyroid cancer is a 'good' cancer had obviously never suffered from it. As of 2019 I am left with a watery and sometimes sore right eye, lymphoedema of the neck, and a tendency for my throat to tighten at the slightest opportunity – but no cancer apart from lung secondaries which do not grow. I hope you've learned something from my experiences, and if you have any questions you can always email me on glenda.shepherd@btconnect.com

Good luck with your own cancer journey!

THE END

If you have enjoyed this book, please consider leaving a review. Thank you. The Coast film is available on the following link: https://www.youtube.com/watch?v=mleaZTXAGug

You can also contact me on my website www.glendashepherd.co.uk
Glenda Shepherd, 2019.

www.ingramcontent.com/pod-product-compliance
Lightning Source LLC
Chambersburg PA
CBHW071556030726
47593CB00001BA/183